THE
BEDSIDE
PALLIATIVE MEDICINE
HANDBOOK

Second Edition

THE
BEDSIDE
PALLIATIVE MEDICINE
HANDBOOK

Second Edition

Editors

Allyn Hum • Neo Han Yee
Poi Choo Hwee • Mervyn Koh

Tan Tock Seng Hospital, Singapore

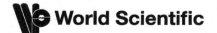
World Scientific

NEW JERSEY • LONDON • SINGAPORE • BEIJING • SHANGHAI • HONG KONG • TAIPEI • CHENNAI • TOKYO

Published by

World Scientific Publishing Co. Pte. Ltd.

5 Toh Tuck Link, Singapore 596224

USA office: 27 Warren Street, Suite 401-402, Hackensack, NJ 07601

UK office: 57 Shelton Street, Covent Garden, London WC2H 9HE

British Library Cataloguing-in-Publication Data
A catalogue record for this book is available from the British Library.

THE BEDSIDE PALLIATIVE MEDICINE HANDBOOK
Second Edition

ISBN 978-981-124-993-8 (hardcover)
ISBN 978-981-125-099-6 (paperback)
ISBN 978-981-124-994-5 (ebook for institutions)
ISBN 978-981-124-995-2 (ebook for individuals)

For any available supplementary material, please visit
https://www.worldscientific.com/worldscibooks/10.1142/12660#t=suppl

Typeset by Stallion Press
Email: enquiries@stallionpress.com

Printed in Singapore

I am indeed honoured to be invited by the editors to pen a few words for this handbook. As we embrace the transformation of Singapore into a first-world society, achieving a 'good death' is increasingly recognised as a medical goal and core competency for the medical profession and its practitioners. Good palliative care in life-limiting conditions goes beyond mere medical treatment; it also includes the psychosocial and ethical aspects of care. It is no longer a bonus, as patients now expect and demand symptomatic relief and optimal pain control.

This handbook, edited by model palliative care specialists Dr Mervyn Koh and Dr Allyn Hum, is therefore a timely addition to the wealth of resources available to local doctors striving to practise good end-of-life care. Unlike many thick encyclopaedias that misleadingly call themselves 'handbooks', this truly lives up to its title — it is small enough to always have on hand.

Full credit should be given to the authors for ensuring the breadth of the contents while keeping the material succinct and user-friendly. The chapter on practical issues in palliative care arms healthcare professionals with much useful information. As a doctor at the front line of care, I am also delighted that this book goes beyond the standard medical treatment to include highly relevant and important topics, such as discussing the extent of care, breaking bad news and advance care planning (ACP).

It is left for me to congratulate the editors and authors on their excellent contribution to palliative care. I am confident that the book will enhance the experience and expertise of healthcare professionals, and ultimately benefit their patients.

Professor Chin Jing Jih
Chairman (Medical Board), Tan Tock Seng Hospital

The Bedside Palliative Care Handbook is a valuable palliative care resource for all healthcare professionals and it is with great anticipation that we welcome this 2nd edition. In addition to the latest updates in palliative care practice, this handbook addresses new areas of Spiritual Care and Ethical Case Analysis, which are critical in our increasingly complex healthcare practice. With palliative care needs set to increase worldwide in the coming years, the 2nd edition of the Bedside Palliative Care Handbook is timely and pertinent. We are grateful to the editors Drs Mervyn Koh, Allyn Hum, Neo Han Yee, Poi Choo Hwee and the contributing authors for sharing their expertise and advancing palliative care education through this handbook.

Dr Patricia Neo Soek Hui
Chairman, Singapore Hospice Council

CONTENTS

ABOUT THE EDITORS

ASSOCIATE PROFESSOR ALLYN HUM

Associate Professor Allyn Hum is a Senior Consultant Geriatrician and Palliative Care Physician at the Department of Palliative Medicine in Tan Tock Seng Hospital.

Currently the Director of the Palliative Care Centre for Excellence in Research and Education (PalC), A/Prof Hum is an advocate of advancing palliative care education through research. Her particular interests include cancer pain and end stage organ disease prognostication.

ASSOCIATE PROFESSOR MERVYN KOH

Associate Professor Mervyn Koh is a Senior Consultant Geriatrician and Palliative Care Physician at the Department of Palliative Medicine in Tan Tock Seng Hospital.

Currently the Medical Director of Dover Park Hospice, A/Prof Koh has advanced knowledge in burnout and resilience in the palliative care community. He attended the Harvard Palliative Care Education Programme and has published book chapters in *Cancer Pain*.

ADJUNCT ASSISTANT PROFESSOR NEO HAN YEE

Dr Neo Han Yee is a Senior Consultant Geriatrician and Head of the Department of Palliative Medicine in Tan Tock Seng Hospital. He has clinical interests in chronic breathlessness and has helped developed integrated palliative rehabilitation programs for patients with advanced lung diseases. Dr Neo also has a keen interest in end-of-life care ethics and currently chairs the Clinical Ethics Committee at Tan Tock Seng Hospital.

ADJUNCT ASSISTANT PROFESSOR POI CHOO HWEE

Dr Poi Choo Hwee is a Senior Consultant with the Department of Palliative Medicine in Tan Tock Seng Hospital (TTSH). She is currently the clinical lead for integrating palliative care in the ICU. She is a Core Clinical Faculty Member of NHG's Internal Medicine Residency Program and site director for Palliative care in the Residency programme at TTSH.

FOREWORD

In this digitalised age where medical information is readily accessible with just a click of a mouse, published guidebooks on clinical practice are still popular among healthcare practitioners. Many practitioners would still prefer to carry around a handy pocket-sized guidebook containing salient information required when faced with an unfamiliar clinical situation.

This handbook on palliative care, the first of its kind published in Singapore and Southeast Asia, comprises a selection of commonly encountered clinical conditions in palliative care with the latest guidelines on its management. Practical issues such as how to facilitate a terminal discharge and where to find community hospices locally are just some of the carefully chosen information included in this handbook. It is, in short, a useful and comprehensive resource to all healthcare workers looking after patients at the end of life or with life-limiting illnesses.

The Bedside Palliative Medicine Handbook is the end product of many hours of research and hard work from a group of dedicated clinicians, nurses and allied health staff from the Palliative Care Department of Tan Tock Seng Hospital and its community partner, Dover Park Hospice. Through this book, we hope to reach out to the healthcare providers caring for the terminally-ill in the course of their work. In doing so, we strive to promote good palliative care for all who need it.

A/Prof Wu Huei Yaw
Deputy Chairman, Medical Board
(Division of Integrated & Community Care)
Woodlands Health

PREFACE

We remember as junior doctors many, many years ago how we had found reader-friendly, succinct and informative handbooks like *The Acute Medicine Handbook* and *The Bedside ICU Handbook* to be invaluable companions in helping to manage our patients.

When we first started out practising palliative care, we struggled to look for a similar handbook which would guide us in managing patients towards the end of life. We also wanted a book which catered to our local palliative care population with drug dosages which would be more appropriate to our patients.

We therefore embarked on an ambitious journey together with our other colleagues in the Department of Palliative Medicine, Tan Tock Seng Hospital as well as Dover Park Hospice to write *The Bedside Palliative Medicine Handbook*, which would provide up-to-date guidelines and recommendations with the aim of helping busy clinicians manage their palliative care patients.

While our recommendations and medication dosages have been researched thoroughly, we do caution that these are also reflective of our institutional practices. Therefore, clinicians should always seek advice from their own primary palliative care provider. The 2nd edition of the Palliative Care Handbook has been updated to include important chapters on ethics, end stage organ disease and community services. Each chapter has also been revised carefully to include current evidence to guide care.

It is our hope that this book will be useful to all clinicians caring for patients with advanced life-limiting illnesses — including House Officers, Residents, Medical Officers, Family Physicians and Senior Clinicians alike. We are also of the opinion that Nurses within all healthcare settings — Acute Hospitals, Home Hospices, Inpatient Hospices, Day Cares, Community Hospitals and Nursing Homes will also find this book helpful.

Allyn Hum, Neo Han Yee, Poi Choo Hwee, Mervyn Koh
Senior Consultants
Department of Palliative Medicine
Tan Tock Seng Hospital

ACKNOWLEDGEMENTS

We would like to thank our colleagues from the Department of Palliative Medicine, Tan Tock Seng Hospital for their valuable contributions to the 2nd edition of the Bedside Palliative Handbook. It is very much a family effort. We are also thankful to Ms Valerie Wu and Ms Jazel Kan for their invaluable administrative support in the production of this book.

A/Prof Wu Huei Yaw has always been a tremendous support and inspiration, and without his encouragement, this book would not have been possible. We would also like to thank our own families who have given us their unconditional love and support in our chosen practice of palliative care.

Our patients and their families have been, and continue to be, our teachers. To them, we owe a great debt of gratitude.

CONTRIBUTORS

Ang Ching Ching
Advanced Practice Nurse
Tan Tock Seng Hospital

Ang Shih-Ling
Principal Resident Physician
Department of Palliative Medicine
Tan Tock Seng Hospital

Aw Chia Hui
Associate Consultant
Palliative and Supportive Care
Department of Integrated Care
Woodlands Health Campus

Chau Mo Yee
Family Physician
Associate Consultant
Department of Palliative Medicine
Tan Tock Seng Hospital

Chen Wei Ting
Advanced Practice Nurse
Tan Tock Seng Hospital

Chia Gerk Sin
Advanced Practice Nurse
Tan Tock Seng Hospital

Chia Siew Chin
Principal Lead (Palliative Medicine)
Lee Kong Chian School of Medicine
Consultant
Department of Palliative Medicine
Tan Tock Seng Hospital

Chiam Zi Yan
Consultant
Department of Palliative Medicine
Tan Tock Seng Hospital

Chong Poh Heng
Medical Director
HCA Hospice Care

Dalisay-Gallardo, Marysol
Resident Physician
Department of Palliative Medicine
Tan Tock Seng Hospital

Goh Wen Yang
Consultant
Department of Palliative Medicine
Tan Tock Seng Hospital

Guan Huey Chen, Jennifer
Associate Consultant
Department of General Medicine
Tan Tock Seng Hospital

Heng Xiaowei
Resident Physician
Palliative and Supportive Care,
Department of Integrated Care
Woodlands Health Campus

Hum Yin Mei, Allyn
Adjunct Associate Professor
Lee Kong Chian School of Medicine
Director
The Palliative Care Centre for Excellence in Research and Education
Senior Consultant
Dover Park Hospice
Department of Palliative Medicine
Tan Tock Seng Hospital

Koh Yong Hwang, Mervyn
Adjunct Associate Professor
Lee Kong Chian School of Medicine
Medical Director
Dover Park Hospice
Senior Consultant
Department of Palliative Medicine
Tan Tock Seng Hospital

Kwan Yunxin
Consultant
Department of Psychiatry
Tan Tock Seng Hospital

Lau Ley Cheng, Joanna
Resident Physician
Department of Palliative Medicine
Tan Tock Seng Hospital

Lee Chung Seng
Consultant
Department of Palliative Medicine
Tan Tock Seng Hospital

Lee Hsien Xiong, Raphael
Clinical Course Lead for OSCE (Clinical Years – Overall)
Lee Kong Chian School of Medicine
Consultant
Palliative and Supportive Care
Department of Integrated Care
Woodlands Health Campus

Lee Hwei Khien
Principal Pharmacist (Clinical)
Tan Tock Seng Hospital

Lim Wen Phei
Assistant Principal Lead (Psychiatry)
Lee Kong Chian School of Medicine
Consultant
Medical Psychiatry, Department of Integrated Care
Woodlands Health Campus

Neo Han Yee
Adjunct Assistant Professor
Clinical Lead (Professionalism, Ethics, Law, Leadership & Patient Safety)
Lee Kong Chian School of Medicine
Head and Senior Consultant
Department of Palliative Medicine
Chairman, Clinical Ethics Committee
Tan Tock Seng Hospital

Ng Han Lip, Raymond
Adjunct Assistant Professor
Lee Kong Chian School of Medicine
Head and Senior Consultant
Palliative and Supportive Care
Department of Integrated Care
Woodlands Health Campus

Ong Wah Ying
Senior Consultant
Division of Supportive and Palliative Care
National Cancer Centre Singapore

Ong Yew Jin, Joseph
Senior Consultant
Dover Park Hospice

Ong Yu Mei, Wendy
Nurse Clinician
Tan Tock Seng Hospital

Poi Choo Hwee
Adjunct Assistant Professor
Lee Kong Chian School of Medicine
Senior Consultant
Department of Palliative Medicine
Tan Tock Seng Hospital

Provido, Mahrley Tanagon
Senior Resident Physician
Department of Palliative Medicine
Tan Tock Seng Hospital

Tan Jiun Yu, Christina
Senior Pharmacist (Clinical)
Tan Tock Seng Hospital

Tham Wai Yong
Psychiatrist

Wiryasaputra, Lynn
Resident Physician
Department of Palliative Medicine
Tan Tock Seng Hospital

Wong Jade Fui
Senior Pharmacist (Clinical)
Tan Tock Seng Hospital

Wu Huei Yaw
Adjunct Associate Professor
Lee Kong Chian School of Medicine
Deputy Chairman
Medical Board (Division of Integrated & Community Care)
Woodlands Health Campus
Senior Consultant
Department of Palliative Medicine
Tan Tock Seng Hospital

Yee Choon Meng
Head of Home Care
Dover Park Hospice
Consultant
Department of Palliative Medicine
Tan Tock Seng Hospital

Yung Sek Hwee, Tricia
Consultant
Department of Palliative Medicine
Tan Tock Seng Hospital

INTRODUCTION

I did not set out to become a palliative care physician. My ambition was to be a family physician; to become the quintessentially wise and beloved family doctor who would grow old together with her patients, with a life spent ministering to generations of families. I seemed to be on track, with my formative years in medicine spent learning how to get patients well and back into the community. Whilst this usually was the case, there remained a population of patients who, in spite of the best physicians and treatment, deteriorated and would eventually die — often in discomfort — leaving behind caregivers, both familial and professional, who questioned if they had done enough. A sense of helplessness was not uncommon during these periods. Little guidance was given as to how best to help the patients and their loved ones in these times of uncertainty and grief.

It appeared that we, as a healthcare community, were more comfortable around the living than we were around the dying. We were denying the possibility of death, even when it became clear that treatment was no longer effective. I puzzled at how we could expect our patients to accept the finality of death when we ourselves talked about it as if it were an affront to medical science that they should die in this medically advanced era. I was certainly not alone in the disquiet I felt when I presented choices to them which were alienating and painful, rather than life-affirming.

It was this disquiet that led me, in my interview to become a medical trainee, to naively tell the interview panel of my decision to eventually "care for the dying", mistakenly naming a specialty I thought would teach me the requisite skills. An eminent member of the panel gently corrected me saying, "… you want to do Palliative Medicine". Even though I had never heard of this field, I thought it best to agree and not look too ignorant.

This was more than 2 decades ago. In the time that I have been training to become a palliative physician, there has been a remarkable growth in the recognition of the need for awareness, knowledge and application of palliative medicine. It is as much a science as it is an art form — the skilful administration of knowledge in a compassionate and caring manner. Appropriately, palliative medicine as a field was officially recognised as a subspecialty in Singapore in 2007.

Although more patients now have access to palliative care at the end of their lives (certainly more than when I first started training), there is undeniably still a gap between the provision of services and the needs of our population, not only in Singapore but globally. The 'silver tsunami' will bring with it an increased prevalence of both malignant and non-malignant maladies as we live longer. Patients, even when living with life-limiting illnesses, have been shown unequivocally to live fulfilling lives when palliative care is introduced. Well-informed treatment decisions can be made with their healthcare providers, and patients can continue living at home or sites of care where they and their families are supported, even up to the time of death. The topic of death is still taboo, but it no longer carries the sense of failure it once did.

In order for our patients to remain comfortable, there needs to be an awareness and acknowledgement that suffering is multi-faceted. For many of our patients and their families, it is comforting for them to know that they are not alone, that they have the support of a multi-disciplinary team, both in the tertiary hospital and within the community. Palliative care challenges have to be met in a variety of settings and this handbook has been written specifically with this aspect in mind.

The multi-disciplinary palliative care team in Tan Tock Seng Hospital and Dover Park Hospice have collaborated to write a handbook that brings together our combined experience in managing the different challenges encountered. Each chapter is written based on the best evidence and research presently available, and can be adapted to any setting of care. The first part of the book focuses on managing symptoms often encountered, be it at home, in the tertiary care setting or inpatient hospice. The second part of the book looks at managing the psychosocial aspects of palliative care, including practical tips at holding difficult conversations with patients and their caregivers. The technical elements of palliative care have also been given their due coverage in this book, including commonly-used medications in palliative care. In this updated edition of the bedside palliative handbook, we have added a substantial section focusing on end stage organ diseases. Our objective for this handbook is to add to the growing body of knowledge in palliative medicine in order for all healthcare providers to be equally adept at caring for patients and their loved ones at the end of life, irrespective of life limiting illness.

Many of us in palliative care are often asked why we practise in this field of medicine, with all its attendant sadness and finality that death brings. My response is invariably "Why not?", especially when I have witnessed how it brings out the very best in medicine and humanity, and where I am learning courage on a daily basis. We, who have the privilege of being called into the healthcare profession, have the opportunity to affirm life, even when life draws to a close, and that, is a blessing indeed.

It is our hope that this book, written with the help of our patients and their families, will be a source of encouragement and practical help to all who have committed themselves to their care.

A/Prof Allyn Hum
December 2021

SECTION 1: PALLIATIVE CARE

WHAT IS PALLIATIVE CARE?

Wu Huei Yaw

Palliative care is an approach which focuses on improving the quality of life of patients suffering from life-limiting illnesses by providing relief from physical, emotional and spiritual suffering. The course of a progressive, incurable illness is marked by a series of losses and challenges. A multi-disciplinary team approach is essential to achieving good care, which includes minimising the impact of the illness and helping patients achieve their personal goals within the limits of their illness.

PRINCIPLES OF PALLIATIVE CARE

The principles of palliative care include:

- Providing relief from distressing symptoms through early identification, assessment and treatment
- Affirming life and regarding dying as a normal process
- Intending neither to hasten nor postpone death
- Integrating the psychosocial, emotional and spiritual aspects into the holistic care of the patient
- Supporting family and caregivers during the patient's illness and after the patient's death

PRINCIPLES OF MANAGEMENT AND DRUG PRESCRIPTION IN PALLIATIVE CARE

The approach to clinical management in palliative care is largely determined by the patient's and family's expectations, the patient's prognosis and goals of care. Although evidence from clinical research has provided useful information, it is important to understand that every patient is different and treatment should be individualised according to the established goals of care.

In palliative medicine, the principles of prescription are uniquely different from other fields of medicine:

- With disease progression, the patient's liver and renal functions are likely to deteriorate. This will have an impact on drug metabolism and elimination. Hence the need to adjust drug dosages accordingly.
- In the terminal stage, many patients are unable to take medication orally and essential medication may have to be switched from the oral route to the parenteral route. The subcutaneous route of drug delivery is preferred because it is relatively easy to administer and less invasive compared to the intravenous or intra-muscular routes.
- Off-label prescription of drugs is not uncommon in palliative care. Many drugs are used because of their positive effects on symptom control. A classic example is the use of Hyoscine Butylbromide (Buscopan) to reduce throat secretions in a terminally-ill patient.

As healthcare providers caring for the terminally-ill, understanding the principles behind palliative management is important in ensuring good care. We hope that this practical bedside handbook will equip the readers with essential information necessary to achieve a level of good palliative care.

SECTION 2: SYMPTOMS

BONE PAIN

Allyn Hum

INTRODUCTION

Bony metastatic disease occurs more commonly than primary bone tumours.

The breasts and lungs are the most common primary disease sites in the female patient, whereas it is the prostate and lungs in the male patient that make up 80% of cancers that spread to the bone.

Skeletal morbidity (skeletal-related events) resulting from metastatic involvement includes:

- Pain
- Hypercalcemia
- Pathological fractures
- Spinal cord or nerve root compression

The most common locations for bony metastatic disease (in order of frequency) are:

- Spine
- Pelvis
- Ribs
- Proximal limb girdles

CAUSES

Pain arising from the cancerous involvement of bone is the commonest cause of cancer-related pain.

Pathophysiological mechanisms:

- Tumour induced osteolysis
- Tumour production of growth factors, cytokines and chemokines
- Neoplastic infiltration of nerves
- Stimulation of ion channels on nociceptive fibres

MANAGEMENT

The use of analgesics according to the WHO Pain Ladder is recommended. NSAIDs and COX-2 Inhibitors are also useful in reducing bone pain.

Radiotherapy (RT)

- Radiotherapy relieves pain in up to 50% of patients and is able to produce complete pain relief in one month in 25% of patients. (NNT to achieve complete pain relief at one month is 4.2). The median duration of complete relief is 12 weeks.
- Single fraction RT is as effective for pain relief as a multi-fractionated schedule
- Use of dexamethasone during RT will reduce bony flare

Radio-pharmaceuticals

- Radio-pharmaceuticals like Strontium are useful for pain control in prostate cancer. The main side-effect is myelosuppression.

Chemotherapy

- Chemotherapy may be useful controlling bone pain by reducing tumour load in chemo-sensitive tumours like multiple myeloma, lymphoma and germ cell tumours.

Orthopaedic Intervention

- Surgical fixation of pathological fractures may be warranted for the relief of pain. Subsequent radiotherapy should also be considered.
- Prophylactic fixation of osteolytic lesions at risk of fracture should also be considered — according to Mirels' Criteria (see below).

Mirels' Criteria (select only one choice per line)

	1	2	3
Site	Upper limb ☐	Lower limb ☐	Peritrochanter ☐
Pain	Mild ☐	Moderate ☐	Severe ☐
Lesion	Osteoblastic ☐	Mixed ☐	Osteolytic ☐
Size	< ⅓ bone diameter ☐	⅓ bone diameter – ⅔ bone diameter ☐	> ⅔ bone diameter ☐

Out of a total score of 12,

- ≤ 7 low risk of fracture
- 8 estimates 15% risk of fracture
- ≥ 9 estimates 33% risk of fracture (Mirels concluded that a score of 9 or greater is an indication for prophylactic fixation)

Bisphosphonates

Used for the relief of bony pain, particularly if pain is present in multiple sites.

- Bisphosphonates should be used in the relief of bone pain if analgesics and radiotherapy are ineffective. NNT is 11 at 4 weeks and 7 at 12 weeks.

- Patients may develop fever and flu-like symptoms subsequently. Osteonecrosis of the jaw is a rare complication.

Bisphosphonate	Intravenous Regime
Pamidronate	• 60–90 mg in 500 ml of N/S over 4 hours
Zoledronic Acid	• 4 mg infused over 15 minutes

RANK-Ligand Inhibitors

- Denosumab reduces the frequency and severity of skeletal related events in cancer
- Evidence of denosumab in the relief of cancer induced bone pain is weak

Interventional Procedures

- Interventional procedures like vertebroplasty or kyphoplasty and nerve blocks should also be considered in patients with refractory pain from pathological fractures or who are intolerant of opioid analgesics.

REFERENCES

1. McQuay HJ, Collins SL, Carroll D, Moore RA, Derry S. Radiotherapy for the palliation of painful bone metastases. *Cochrane Database Syst Rev.* 2013;2013(11):CD001793.
2. Rich SE, Chow R, Chow E, *et al.* Update of the systematic review of palliative radiation therapy fractionation for bone metastases. *Radiat Oncol.* 2018 March;126(3):547–557.
3. Mirels H. Metastatic disease in long bones. *Clin Orthop Relat Res.* 1989;249: 256–264.
4. Porta-Sales J, Garzón-Rodríguez C, Caraceni A, *et al.* Evidence on the analgesic role of bisphosphonates and denosumab in the treatment of pain due to bone metastases: A systematic review within the European Association for Palliative Care guidelines project. *Palliat Med.* 2017 Jan;31(1):5–25.

BRAIN METASTASIS

Ong Wah Ying and Marysol Dalisay-Gallardo

INTRODUCTION

Brain metastasis is the most common intracranial tumour in adults. 10–20% of cancer patients will develop symptomatic brain metastasis. Commonly involved intracranial sites include the cerebral hemispheres (80%), cerebellum (15%) and the brainstem (5%). There are usually multiple metastases upon diagnosis.

CLINICAL PRESENTATION

Headache, vomiting, neurological deficits, seizures, altered mental state, cognitive impairment (up to 65%)

CAUSES

The common cancers that metastasize to the brain include:

- Lung cancer
- Breast cancer
- Malignant Melanoma
- Kidney cancer
- GIT

PROGNOSTICATION

Prognostication in brain metastasis is increasingly individualized by cancer type and molecular genetic diagnosis.

Diagnosis-Specific Graded Prognostic Assessment (GPA)

Breast Cancer

Prognostic Factor	GPA Score					Patient Score
	0	0.5	1.0	1.5	2.0	
KPS	≤60	70–80	90–100	NA	NA	
Age	≥60	<60	NA	NA	NA	
No. of BM	≥2	1	NA	NA	NA	
ECM	Present	Absent	NA	NA	NA	
Subtype	Basal	Luminal A	NA	Her2 or Luminal B	NA	
					Sum:	

Sum = Median survival (months) by GPA: 0 – 1 = 6; 1.5 – 2.0 = 13; 2.5 – 3.0 = 24; 3.5 – 4.0 = 36
Basal: triple negative (ER/PR/HER2–); Luminal A (ER/PR+, HER2–); Luminal B (triple positive, ER/PR/HER2+); HER2 (HER2+, ER/PR–)

NSCLC Adenocarcinoma

Prognostic Factor	GPA Score					Patient Score
	0	0.5	1.0	1.5	2.0	
KPS	≤70	80	90–100	NA	NA	
Age	≥70	<70	NA	NA	NA	
No. of BM	≥5	1–4	NA	NA	NA	
ECM	Present	NA	Absent	NA	NA	
EGFR and ALK	Both neg or unknown	NA	EGFR or ALK positive	NA	NA	
					Sum:	

Sum = Median survival (months) by GPA: 0 – 1 = 7; 1.5 – 2.0 = 13; 2.5 – 3.0 = 25; 3.5 – 4.0 = 46

NSCLC Non-Adenocarcinoma

Prognostic Factor	GPA Score					Patient Score
	0	0.5	1.0	1.5	2.0	
KPS	≤70	80	90–100	NA	NA	
Age	≥70	<70	NA	NA	NA	
No. of BM	≥5	1–4	NA	NA	NA	
ECM	Present	NA	Absent	NA	NA	
					Sum:	

Sum = Median survival (months) by GPA: 0 – 1 = 5; 1.5 – 2.0 = 10; 2.5 – 3.0 = 13; 3.5 – 4.0 = NA

Renal Cell Carcinoma

Prognostic Factor	GPA Score					Patient Score
	0	0.5	1.0	1.5	2.0	
KPS	≤70	NA	80	NA	90–100	
No. of BM	≥5,	1–4	NA	NA	NA	
ECM	Present	Absent	NA	NA	NA	
Hgb	<11.1	11.1–12.5 or unknown	>12.5	NA	NA	
					Sum:	

Sum = Median survival (months) by GPA: 0 – 1 = 4; 1.5 – 2.0 = 12; 2.5 – 3.0 = 17; 3.5 – 4.0 = 35

Melanoma

Prognostic Factor	GPA Score					Patient Score
	0	0.5	1.0	1.5	2.0	
KPS	≤70	80	90–100	NA	NA	
Age	≥70	<70	NA	NA	NA	
No. of BM	≥5	2–4	1	NA	NA	
ECM	Present	NA	Absent	NA	NA	
BRAF	Negative or unknown	Positive	NA	NA	NA	
					Sum:	

Sum = Median survival (months) by GPA: 0 – 1 = 5; 1.5 – 2.0 = 8; 2.5 – 3.0 = 16; 3.5 – 4.0 = 34

Gastrointestinal Cancers

Prognostic Factor	GPA Score					Patient Score
	0	0.5	1.0	1.5	2.0	
KPS	≤70	NA	80	NA	90–100	
Age	≥60	<60	NA	NA	NA	
No. of BM	≥4	2–3	1			
ECM	Present	Absent	NA	NA	NA	
					Sum:	

Sum = Median survival (months) by GPA: 0 – 1 = 3; 1.5 – 2.0 = 7; 2.5 – 3.0 = 11; 3.5 – 4.0 = 17

Abbreviation: BM, brain metastases; ECM, extracranial metastases; Hgb, hemoglobin; KPS, Karnofsky performance status; NSCLC, non–small-cell lung cancer.

TREATMENT

Role of Surgery

- Surgery + Whole Brain Radiotherapy (WBRT) is recommended as 1st line treatment in patients with single brain metastases with favourable performance status and limited extracranial disease to extend overall/median survival and local control. (Level 1 recommendation)
- Surgery + Stereotactic Radiosurgery (SRS) is recommended to provide survival benefit in patients with metastatic brain tumours. (Level 3 recommendation)
- In patients with multiple brain metastases, tumour resection is recommended in patients with lesions inducing symptoms from mass effect that can be reached without inducing new neurological deficits and who have control of their cancer outside the nervous system. (Level 3 recommendation)

Role of WBRT

- Can improve progression-free survival for patients with >4 brain metastases (Level 3 recommendation)
  - Standard WBRT dose is 30 Gy in 10 fractions (Level 1 recommendation)
  - 20 Gy in 5 fractions is for patients with poor performance status or short predicted survival (Level 3 recommendation)
  - Patients having WBRT should be offered 6 months of memantine to potentially delay, lessen, or prevent the associated neurocognitive toxicity
- Due to neurocognitive toxicity, local therapy [surgery or (SRS)] without WBRT is recommended for patients with ≤4 brain metastases amenable to local therapy. (Level 2 recommendation)
- WBRT after surgery or SRS is not recommended in patients with WHO performance status 0–2 and with up to 4 brain metastases because it does not improve overall survival. (Level 2 recommendation)
  - The addition of WBRT after surgery or SRS is also not recommended for patients with >4 brain metastases unless the metastases' volume exceeds 7 ml or there are >15 metastases, or the size or location of the metastases are not amenable to surgical resection or radiosurgery (Level 3 recommendation)
- Although prophylactic cranial irradiation (PCI) decreases the risk of brain metastases in both limited and extensive small-cell lung cancer, its role in improving survival is less clear. Its use should be adapted to risk.

Role of SRS

- Alternative to surgical resection in solitary brain metastasis when surgical resection is likely to induce new neurological deficits and tumour volume and location are not likely to be associated with radiation-induced injury to surrounding structures (Level 3 recommendation)
- Should be used to decrease local recurrence rates after surgery of solitary brain metastasis (Level 3 recommendation)

- Recommended for patients with 2–4 brain metastases or even those with >4 metastases, if the cumulative metastases volume is <7ml (Level 3 recommendation)

Role of Systemic Chemotherapy/Molecular Targeted Agents/Immunotherapy

- Routine use of cytotoxic chemotherapy alone for brain metastases is not recommended as it has not been shown to increase overall survival. (Level 1 recommendation)
- Routine use of chemotherapy following WBRT or SRS for brain metastases is not recommended. (Level 1 recommendation)
- The role of immunotherapy and molecular targeted agents for brain metastases are evolving and have begun to offer greater potential for certain types of cancer.

Supportive Care

- For patients with poor performance status and progressive systemic disease, best supportive care may be more appropriate.

SYMPTOM MANAGEMENT

- Corticosteroids are used to control vasogenic oedema. The recommended dose of dexamethasone is between 4–16 mg/day in divided doses (PO/IV).
- Available data support recommendation against the routine use of prophylactic anticonvulsants in brain metastasis patients without prior history of seizures, both in nonsurgical and post-operative settings.
  - For management of seizures, avoid enzyme-inducing antiepileptic drugs and consider as first-choice newer generation drugs like Levetiracetam.
- Anticoagulation with either LMWH or DOACs should be considered in patients with venous thromboembolism and brain metastasis.

REFERENCES

1. Sperduto PW, *et al*. Survival in patients with brain metastases: Summary report on the updated diagnosis-specific graded prognostic assessment and definition of the eligibility quotient. *J Clin Oncol*. 2020;38(32):3773–3784.
2. Ammirati M, *et al*. Congress of neurological surgeons systematic review and evidence-based guidelines on treatment options for adults with multiple metastatic brain tumors. *Neurosurgery*. 2019;84:E180–E182.
3. Ryken TC, *et al*. Congress of neurological surgeons systematic review and evidence-based guidelines on the role of steroids in the treatment of adults with metastatic brain tumors. *Neurosurgery*. 2019;84:E189–E191.
4. Chen C, *et al*. Congress of neurological surgeons systematic review and evidence-based guidelines on the role of prophylactic anticonvulsants in the treatment of adults with metastatic brain tumors. *Neurosurgery*. 2019;84: E195–E197.
5. Mulvenna P, *et al*. Dexamethasone and supportive care with or without whole brain radiotherapy in treating patients with non-small cell lung cancer with brain metastases unsuitable for resection or stereotactic radiotherapy (QUARTZ): results from a phase 3, non-inferiority, randomised trial. *Lancet*. 2016;388:2004–2014.
6. Carney BJ, *et al*. Intracranial hemorrhage with direct oral anticoagulants in patients with brain tumors. *J Thromb Haemost*. 2019;17:72–76.

CANCER PAIN

Allyn Hum and Raphael Lee

INTRODUCTION

"Hope is the physician of each misery."

— *Irish Proverb*

Pain is one of the most feared consequences of cancer, associated with intolerable suffering, both physical and emotional.

Pain is present in almost 24–62% of patients at the time of diagnosis and in almost all patients at the terminal stages of illness.

A significant proportion of patients still live with disabling pain despite advances in the understanding of cancer pain management.

ASSESSMENT OF CANCER PAIN

"Pain is what the patient says it is, and exists whenever he or she says it does."

— *Margo McCaffery*

The optimal management of pain is dependent on the patient's description of their experience.

1. Temporal pattern (onset, pattern and course)
2. Location
3. Pattern of radiation
4. Intensity of pain (verbal rating scale, numerical rating scale)

5. Type of pain (nociceptive descriptors, neuropathic descriptors)
6. Relieving and aggravating precipitants
7. Analgesia history
8. Impact of pain on function
9. Impact of pain on mood, psycho-emotional state and quality of life

CATEGORIES OF CANCER PAIN

'Physiological' pain categories:

Type of Pain	Example	Mechanism
Nociceptive Somatic Pain	• Neoplastic invasion of bone, joint, muscle or connective tissue	Activation of nociceptors
Nociceptive Visceral Pain	• Obstruction, infiltration or compression of visceral organs	Activation of nociceptors
Neuropathic Pain	• Neoplastic infiltration or compression of nerve, plexus or roots	Direct injury or dysfunction of the somatosensory nervous system

MANAGEMENT

- Disease modifying treatment, i.e. palliative radiotherapy, chemotherapy, surgery
- Identify psychosocial/emotional/spiritual triggers
- Change route of administration of opioids
- Opioid rotation
- Use of adjuvants
- Interventional analgesic techniques
- Education of patient about pain and its management so they can play an active role

PHARMACOLOGICAL APPROACH TO CANCER PAIN MANAGEMENT

WHO Pain Ladder: By the clock, round the clock

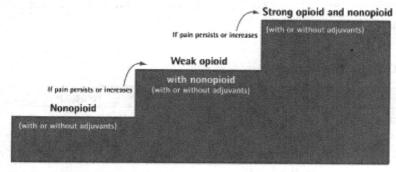

Adapted from the World Health Organization.[1]

Fig. 1: The World Health Organization analgesic ladder for treating cancer pain

Modification of the WHO Pain Ladder

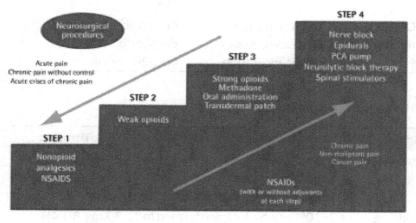

NSAID—nonsteroidal anti-inflammatory drug; PCA—patient-controlled analgesia.

Fig. 2: New adaptation of the analgesic ladder

Analgesics on the pain ladder are administered based on the intensity and frequency of pain ie therapeutics need not be escalated strictly step by step to target severe pain and can start at the highest step

As with adjuvants, interventional techniques can help at any step of the pain ladder, and may not necessarily be reserved only for use at the 4th step.

WHO Step 1 Medications

Agent	Mechanism of Action	Titration
Paracetamol	• Weak prostaglandin inhibitor • Primarily metabolised in the liver	2–4 g/day
NSAIDs	• Inhibit Cyclooxygenase 1 & 2 • Antipyretic and anti-inflammatory	Ibuprofen 400 mg TDS Naproxen 250–500 mg BD Diclofenac 50 mg BD-TDS (Suppository form: 25–50 mg TDS)
COX-2 Inhibitors	• Anti-inflammatory • Decreased risk of peptic ulceration	Celecoxib 200 mg BD Etoricoxib 60–120 mg OM

WHO Step 2 Medications

Agent	Mechanism of Action	Titration
Tramadol	• Weak μ-opioid receptor agonist • Inhibits serotonin and noradrenaline reuptake	25–50 mg q8H (max: 400 mg/day)
Codeine Phosphate	• 2–10% will be biotransformed to Morphine	30 mg BD-4H (max: q4H)

WHO Step 3 Medications

Agent (Immediate Release)	Mechanism of Action	Titration
Morphine solution	• μ-opioid receptor agonists	2.5 mg q4H
Oxycodone/Oxynorm	• μ-opioid, k-opioid agonists	5 mg q4H
Methadone	• μ-opioid, ∂-opioid agonists	Specialist
	• NMDA receptor antagonist	review

Agent (Controlled Release)	Mechanism of Action	Titration
Morphine Sulphate Tab	• μ-opioid agonist	10 mg q12H
Oxycontin	• μ-opioid agonist	10 mg q12H
Transdermal Fentanyl	• μ-opioid agonist	12 mcg/hr q72H

Adjuvant Analgesics

Helpful in neuropathic pain; can be added at **any step** of the WHO Pain Ladder

Agent	Mechanism of Action	Titration
Antidepressants		
TCAs	• Na channel blockers • Inhibits reuptake of serotonin and norepinephrine	Nortriptylline 10–100 mg ON Amitriptyline 10–75 mg ON
SNRIs	• Inhibits reuptake of serotonin and norepinephrine	Duloxetine 30–60 mg OM Venlafaxine 37.5 mg – 150 mg OD
Anticonvulsants		
Gabapentin	• Ca channel blocker • Decreases release of glutamate and substance P	100–300 mg OD-TDS (max: 3600 mg/day)
Pregabalin	• Ca channel blocker • Decreases release of glutamate and substance P	75–150 mg OD-BD (max: 600 mg/day)

Agent	Mechanism of Action	Titration
Anaesthetics		
Lignocaine (topical)	Na channel blocker Mechanical allodynia	5% patch OD (for 12 hrs) (max: 3 patches/day)
Lignocaine (parenteral)	Na channel blocker	Test dose of 2 mg/kg Infusion of 1–2 mg/kg/hr
Ketamine	NMDA receptor antagnonist	75–475 mg/day
Steroids		
Dexamethasone	• Anti-inflammatory	4–8 mg OD

REFERENCES

1. Bruera E, Kin HN. Cancer pain. *JAMA*. 2003;290(18):2476–2479.
2. Cleary J. The pharmacological management of cancer pain. *J Palliat Med*. 2007;10:1369–1395.
3. Finnerup ND, Otto M, McQuay HJ. Algorithm for neuropathic pain control: An evidence based proposal. *Pain*. 2005;118(3):289–305.
4. Chapman EJ, Edwards Z, Boland JW, *et al.* Practice review: Evidence-based and effective management of pain in patients with advanced cancer. *Palliat Med*. 2020;34(4):444–453.
5. WHO Guidelines for the pharmacological and radiotherapeutic management of cancer pain in adults and adolescents. *Geneva: World Health Organization*; 2018. Licence. CC BY-NC-SA 3.0 ICO.

CONSTIPATION

Raymond Ng and Chen Wei Ting

INTRODUCTION

Constipation is a highly prevalent and distressing symptom in many patients with cancer, chronic illness and advanced age. It is a common adverse effect associated with opioids.

Generally, constipation may be a problem if a patient is defecating less than three times per week. It is primarily associated with infrequent (relative to the patient's normal bowel habits) and difficult passage of small, hard stools. Other symptoms include the inability to defecate at will, discomfort when defecating, unproductive urge and straining, bloating and a sensation of incomplete evacuation.

Always elucidate the underlying causes through history, physical examination and appropriate investigations. Prevent the onset of constipation through judicious advice and use of laxatives.

CAUSES

Drugs	• Opioids
	• Tricyclic antidepressants
	• Ondansetron
	• Calcium supplements
	• Iron supplements

Metabolic	• Dehydration • Hypercalcemia • Hypokalemia • Hypothyroidism • Diabetes mellitus • Uraemia
Neurological	• Parkinson's Disease • Brain tumours • Spinal cord compression • Autonomic dysfunction • Sacral nerve infiltration
Structural	• Gastrointestinal or pelvic tumours • Peritoneal metastasis • Adhesions
Pain	• Anal fissures • Haemorrhoids
Psychological	• Lack of privacy or comfort because of assistance with toileting, reduced mobility, depression, sedation

MANAGEMENT

Non-Pharmacological

- Ensure adequate fluid intake with increased consumption of high water content foods such as soups, yogurt and fortified supplements
- Not advisable to encourage increase in fibre intake in the elderly and patients on palliative care, especially when fluid consumption is less than 1.5 L per day
- Encourage patient mobility
- Encourage toileting in the morning 20 minutes after breakfast because of the powerful gastro-colic reflex
- Maintain privacy and avoid bedpans if possible (as bedpans inhibit privacy and make it difficult for patients to generate enough intra-abdominal pressure)

Pharmacological — Commonly Used Drugs

It is common practice to combine the use of an osmotic laxative together with a colonic (peristaltic) stimulant, e.g. Lactulose 10 ml TDS and Senna 2 tabs ON.

Osmotic laxatives

- Lactulose 10-20 ml BD-TDS
    — May cause flatulence or abdominal distension
- Forlax 1 sachet OM-TDS
    — May cause diarrhoea
- Polyethylene Glycol (PEG) 1 sachet (dilute to 1 litre)
    — Usually only used for bowel preparation before endoscopy as it can cause profuse diarrhoea
- Fleet (Saline) and Centa Enema x 1
    — Given per rectally
    — Avoid fleet enema in patients with renal failure due to high phosphate content

Colonic Stimulants

- Senna (peristaltic stimulant) 2 tabs ON-TDS
    — May cause abdominal cramps

Rectal Stimulants

- Bisacodyl (Dulcolax) suppository 1-2 supps (10 mg each) OM
    — May cause abdominal cramps

Oral Prolonged-Release Oxycodone/Naloxone *(only for Opioid-Induced Constipation)*

- Prolonged-release Oxycodone/Naloxone tablets 5 mg/2.5 mg (lowest dose)
    — Duration of action is 12 hours
    — Daily starting dose is titrated based on opioid requirements

— Can be used when other causes of constipation have been excluded and opioids determined as the main cause
— Oral Naloxone has low oral bioavailability and will not reduce the analgesic effect of opioids

PRACTICAL TIPS

1. Exclude bowel obstruction, spurious or overflow diarrhoea. Where needed, perform further imaging studies such as an abdominal X-ray.
2. Treat related symptoms such as nausea and vomiting.
3. Oral laxatives are used in preference to rectal treatments. Rectal medications are used in patients who cannot consume orally, have faecal impaction, or suffer with spinal cord lesions and denervation of the colon.
4. In patients with spinal cord compression, avoid osmotic laxatives which may lead to overly soft stools that can cause skin rash and excoriation. Use stimulants instead.
5. Bulking agents are not recommended in palliative patients due to reduced fluid intake when they become more ill.
6. Minimise drugs causing constipation but do not decrease opioids unless absolutely necessary as it may aggravate pain or breathlessness. In general, prescribe laxatives prophylactically with opioids.
7. Patients using oral oxycodone/naloxone formulations may still require laxatives to address constipation if severe.

REFERENCES

1. Librach SL, Bouvette M. Consensus recommendations for the management of constipation in patients with advanced, progressive illness. *J Pain Symptom Manage.* 2010;40(5):761–773.
2. Larkin PJ, Sykes NP. The management of constipation in palliative care: Clinical practice recommendations. *Palliat Med.* 2008;22(7):796–807.
3. Morlion BJ, *et al.* Oral prolonged-release Oxycodone/Naloxone for management pain and opioid induced constipation: A review of the evidence. *Clin Drug Investig.* 2017;37(12):1191–1201.

DELIRIUM

Mervyn Koh and Ang Shih-Ling

Mervyn Koh and Ang Shih-Ling

INTRODUCTION

Delirium occurs commonly (up to 88%) in patients near the end of life. It is a poor prognostic indicator and is associated with high mortality. Three forms of delirium are commonly encountered: Hyperactive, Hypoactive and Mixed Delirium. It is purported to be due to the inhibition of acetylcholine pathways and excess dopaminergic stimulation.

CLINICAL FEATURES

Diagnosis can be made with the CAM (Confusion Assessment Method). It should fulfil the following criteria (1 + 2, plus either 3 or 4):
1. Acute onset and fluctuating course
2. Inattention
    - Difficulty focusing attention, being easily distractible or having difficulty keeping track of what was being said
3. Clouded consciousness
    - Ranging from hyperalert to stuporous
4. Disorganised thinking
    - Rambling or irrelevant conversation, unclear or illogical flow of ideas, or unpredictable switching from subject to subject

CAUSES

The causes of delirium can be easily remembered with the mnemonic – DELIRIUM. It is important to note that up to 50% of these causes are reversible.

Drugs	• Anti-cholinergic drugs • Steroids • Opioids • Tricyclic antidepressants (TCA)
Electrolytes	• Hypercalcemia • Hypoglycemia • Hypernatremia • Hyponatremia
Lung/Liver	• Pneumonia • Pulmonary embolism • Hepatic encephalopathy
Infections	• Consider possible infection sites
Retention/Restraints	• Urinary retention • Faecal impaction • Use of restraints
Intracranial	• Brain metastasis • Stroke • Seizures
Uraemia	• Renal failure
Myocardial	• Myocardial infarction

Note: Of the above, the common reversible causes to look out for include drugs, infections and electrolyte imbalance.

MANAGEMENT

Pharmacological

First Line
- Haloperidol (drops/tablets) 0.5–1.5 mg QDS
- Risperidone (drops/tablets) 0.5–1.0 mg TDS

(For patients with Parkinson's disease or who develop extra-pyramidal side-effects with Haloperidol)

Second Line
If the patient is still agitated despite the above, consider:
- Oral (PO) or Sublingual Lorazepam 0.5–1.0 mg ON
- Switching from Haloperidol to oral or sublingual Olanzapine 2.5 mg OD-TDS
- Chlorpromazine 12.5–50 mg ON

PRACTICAL TIPS

For patients who are very agitated and refuse to take oral medications, consider using:
1. SC Haloperidol 1.0–2.5 mg stat (not more than 10 mg per day)
2. SC Midazolam 1.0–2.5 mg stat (for anxiety)
3. SC Midazolam infusion starting at 0.2 mg/hr to control refractory agitated delirium.

Non-Pharmacological

1. Minimise the use of catheters, intravenous lines and physical restraints
2. Minimize excessive noise
3. Avoid immobility and promote early mobilisation
4. Monitor nutrition and prevent dehydration
5. Optimise pain control
6. Monitor bowel and bladder function
7. Review medications

REFERENCES

1. Breitbart W, Alici Y. Agitation and delirium towards the end of life: 'We couldn't manage him'. *JAMA*. 2008;300(24):2898–2910.
2. Caraceni A, Simonetti F. Palliating delirium in patients with cancer. *Lancet Oncol*. 2009;10:164–172.

3.   Bush SH, Currow DC, Bruera E. Treating an established episode of delirium in palliative care: Expert opinion and a review of the current evidence base with recommendations for future development. *J Pain Symptom Manage.* Aug 2014;8(2):231–247.

DIARRHOEA

Mervyn Koh and Ang Shih-Ling

INTRODUCTION

Diarrhoea is a common symptom that occurs in palliative care patients. It causes them significant distress and can lead to dehydration, electrolyte imbalance, malnutrition and pressure ulcers.

DEFINITION

Diarrhoea is defined as the passage of >3 episodes of unformed stools in a day. Another classification system is the National Cancer Institute's Common Terminology Criteria for Adverse Events (CTCAE) for diarrhoea severity which describes treatment-related diarrhoea:

Grade 1	• Increase of < 4 stools /day over over baseline
Grade 2	• Increase of 4–6 stools /day over baseline
Grade 3	• Increase of ≥7 stools/day over baseline
Grade 4	• Life-threatening consequences; urgent intervention indicated

CAUSES

There are multiple causes of diarrhoea. The first step is always to exclude 'Spurious Diarrhoea', either from the over-use of laxatives or from constipation and faecal impaction.

1. General Causes of Diarrhoea

- Gastroenteritis
  - Viruses and common bacteria such as *E. coli, Campylobacter* and *Salmonella*
- *Clostridium difficile* (*C. diff.*)
  - Cancer patients are prone to *C. diff.* infections as they are immuno-compromised and often receive multiple broad-spectrum antibiotics (especially penicillins and cephalosporins)
  - Specific treatment is with oral metronidazole 400 mg TDS for 10 days or oral vancomycin 125 mg every 6 hourly (if severe)
- Enteral feeding
  - Tube-feeding can cause diarrhoea in 10–60% of patients due to the high osmotic content, rapid or high volume feeding and hypoalbuminemia
  - Switching to higher fibre feeds like Jevity may help
- Tumour-related causes
  - Rectal cancers commonly secrete mucus that may present as diarrhoea
  - Pancreatic cancer causing pancreatic or biliary obstruction can cause diarrhoea
  - May use Creon (pancrelipase), which is a pancreatic enzyme, with a proton pump inhibitor and titrate doses based on symptom relief (oral pancrelipase 25,000–50,000 units/meal but not more than 2500 units/kg/meal)
  - Rare causes include VIPomas (Vaso-active intestinal peptide) and gastrinomas

2. Treatment-Related Causes

- Chemotherapy-related
  - Chemotherapy destroys intestinal epithelial crypt cells and leads to villous sloughing, which results in poorer absorption and increased intestinal secretions
  - Common chemotherapy drugs like 5-Fluorouracil (5-FU) and its prodrug Capecitabine, Irinotecan and Docetaxel have all been implicated in causing diarrhoea
  - Targeted therapy drugs like Erlotinib, Gefitinib, Imatinib, Sorafenib and Sunitinib also cause diarrhoea
  - Neutropenic Enterocolitis occurs when Absolute Neutrophil Count (ANC) is <500/μL, where patients present with fever, abdominal pain and diarrhoea. The risk of mortality is high.
- Radiotherapy-related
  - Acute Radiation Enterocolitis
    i) Occurs within the first six weeks of radiotherapy to the abdomen or pelvis
    ii) Radiotherapy causes increased prostaglandin secretion and reduced bile re-absorption leading to diarrhoea
    iii) Diarrhoea may be associated with tenesmus and bleeding and may take weeks to months to resolve
  - Chronic Radiation Enterocolitis
    i) Occurs months to years after radiotherapy, usually associated with fractions >45 Gy and is due to radiation endarteritis leading to ischaemia and malabsorption
- Post-surgical/post-procedural
  - Patients who have had Whipple's surgery and gastrectomy, or in whom >100 cm of ileum resected are prone to diarrhoea
  - Extensive colectomy causes reduced water absorption and diarrhoea
  - Coeliac plexus block can lead to loss of sympathetic tone and acute diarrhoea

MANAGEMENT

Non-Pharmacological

- Exclude causes of 'spurious diarrhoea'
- Change to a non-milk diet
- Use oral rehydration salts or isotonic drinks
- Replace electrolytes lost due to hyponatremia or hypokalemia
- Prevent pressure ulcers with barrier creams, pressure-relief mattresses and regular turning

Pharmacological

- Loperamide 2-4 mg TDS (up to maximum 16 mg/day)
  — An opioid agonist which acts only locally on the myenteric plexus of the colon and is minimally absorbed
- Hyoscine Butylbromide (Buscopan) 20 mg BD-TDS
  — It can be added if Loperamide is ineffective
- Codeine Phosphate 30 mg TDS-QDS can also be used
- Octreotide (Somatostatin analogue) SC as an infusion 300 mcg/day
  — If the patient does not improve, adding Loperamide and Hyoscine Butylbromide is helpful

PRACTICAL TIP

1. Avoid Lomotil (Diphenoxylate/Atropine) in the elderly as Atropine may cause delirium.

REFERENCES

1. Cherny N. Evaluation and management of treatment-related diarrhoea in patients with advanced cancer: A review. *J Pain Symptom Manage.* 2008;36(4):413–423.
2. Alderman J. Diarrhoea in palliative care. *J Palliat Med.* 2005;8(2):449–450.
3. Bossi P, *et al*. Diarrhoea in adult cancer patients: ESMO clinical practice guidelines. *Ann Oncol.* 2018;29(Suppl 4): iv126–iv142.
4. Common Terminology Criteria for Adverse Events (CTCAE), Version 5.0, November 2017, National Institutes of 4. Health, National Cancer Institute. Available at: https://ctep.cancer.gov/protocoldevelopment/electronic_applications/docs/CTCAE_v5_Quick_Reference_8.5x11.pdf

DYSPNEA

Mervyn Koh and Ang Shih-Ling

INTRODUCTION

Dyspnea is a subjective 'feeling of breathlessness' experienced commonly by patients with cancers (up to 90% in lung cancer) and end-stage organ failure (75% in COLD-SUPPORT Study).

It often causes significant distress and anxiety in patients and their loved ones.

As in cancer pain, many patients with dyspnea also have a 'steady' state with episodes of 'breakthrough' dyspnea which often occurs during movement or at night. While other symptoms like pain, nausea and vomiting may improve towards the end-of-life, dyspnea usually does not and may even worsen.

The severity of dyspnea can be assessed by the Numeric Rating Scale (NRS).

CAUSES

Common conditions that cause dyspnea can be cancer-related, treatment-related or due to existing co-morbidities.

1. Cancer-related causes can be further classified into:
   - Lung: Tumour obstruction, pleural effusion or post-obstructive pneumonia
   - Cardiovascular: Pulmonary embolism, SVCO or pericardial effusion

- Lymphatics: Lymphangitis Carcinomatosis
- Extrinsic Compression: Mediastinal lymphadenopathy, diaphragmatic splinting (Gross Ascites/Hepatomegaly)
2. Treatment-related causes:
   - Chemotherapy induced pneumonitis
   - Radiation induced pneumonitis
   - Doxorubicin-induced cardiomyopathy
3. Co-morbidities:
   - COPD, interstitial lung disease
   - Heart Failure
   - Anaemia

Note: The more common causes of dyspnea in cancer patients are pneumonia, pleural effusion, pulmonary embolism, COPD exacerbation and heart failure.

MANAGEMENT

Treat the Underlying Cause

- Pleural drainage for symptomatic pleural effusion
- Antibiotics for pneumonia
- Stenting an obstructed airway

Pharmacological (titrate to effect)

- Mist Morphine 2.5–5 mg 4–6 hourly (Mild to Moderate Dyspnea)
- Parenteral Infusions: Morphine 0.2–1 mg/hr (Moderate to Severe Dyspnea)
- Alprazolam 0.25–0.5 mg TDS PRN (anxiety) and/or Lorazepam 0.5–1 mg ON PRN for insomnia

Non-Pharmacological

- Supplemental oxygen is beneficial for hypoxic patients
- Blowing cool air (via fan) on the face may be useful for relieving dyspnea by stimulating the trigeminal nerve

- Cognitive Behavioural Therapy, which combines the approach of breathing retraining, exercise, counselling, relaxation, coping and adaptation strategies may improve breathlessness

PRACTICAL TIPS

1. A significant proportion (almost 50%) of patients with dyspnea also experience anxiety and insomnia. It is good practice to ask for these associated symptoms in any dyspnoeic patient.
2. There is often a strong psychological component that influences or aggravates dyspnea. Therefore, it is important to combine both pharmacological and non-pharmacological measures to manage dyspnea.

REFERENCES

1. Luce JM, Luce JA. Management of dyspnea in patients with far-advanced lung disease. *JAMA*. 2001;285(210):1331–1337.
2. DiSalvo WM, Joyce MM, *et al.* Putting evidence into practice. Evidence-based intervention for cancer-related dyspnea. *Clini J Oncol Nurs.* April 2008;12(2):341–352.
3. Mark B. Parshall *et al.* An official American Thoracic Society Statement: Update on the mechanisms, assessment and management of dyspnea. *Am J Respir Crit Med.* 2012;185:435–450.
4. Barnes H, McDonald J, *et al.* Opioids for the palliation of refractory breathlessness in adults with advanced disease and terminal illness. *Cochrane Database Syst Rev.* 2016;3:Cdo11008

HICCUPS

Allyn Hum and Marysol Dalisay-Gallardo

INTRODUCTION

Hiccups are caused by the repeated, involuntary, spasmodic contraction of the diaphragm and inspiratory muscles, followed by sudden closure of the glottis.

The incidence of hiccups is unknown in the terminally ill but if persistent, can be a distressing symptom to both patients and caregivers.

CATEGORIES OF HICCUPS

Hiccups can be categorised by their duration.

Hiccup Bout	• <48 hours
Persistent Hiccups	• >48 hours but <1 month
Intractable Hiccups	• >1 month

PATHOPHYSIOLOGY

The hiccup reflex comprises:

Afferent Limb	• Phrenic and vagus nerves and sympathetic chain (T6–12)
Hiccup Centres	• Hypothalamus, Medulla, Brainstem and Cervical spinal cord (C3–5)
Efferent Limbs	• Phrenic nerve causing the contraction of the diaphragm and intercostal muscles • Recurrent laryngeal nerve causing glottis closure

CAUSES OF PERSISTENT HICCUPS

Can be broadly divided into central, peripheral (gastrointestinal and non-gastrointestinal) and other causes. These respond differently to pharmacological interventions.

Central Cause	Common Conditions
Neurological	Cerebrovascular accident, multiple sclerosis, parkinsonism, brain tumours and metastases, meningitis, encephalitis
Non-neurological	Infection, trauma

Peripheral Cause	Common Conditions
Gastrointestinal	Distension, gastro-oesophageal reflux disease, gastritis, peptic ulcer disease, pancreatitis, gallbladder disease, hepatitis, aerophagia, bowel obstruction, neoplasm
Non-gastrointestinal	Thoracic (myocardial infarction, pericarditis, aortic aneurysm, pneumonia, bronchitis, tuberculosis), neoplasm, rhinitis, otitis, pharyngitis

Other causes	Common Examples
Toxic metabolic	Alcohol, diabetes, systemic infections (influenza, tuberculosis, malaria), hyponatraemia, hypokalaemia, hypocalcaemia, hypocapnia, uraemia

(*Continued*)	
Drugs	Opioids, diazepam, barbiturates, dexamethasone, alpha-methyldopa, dopamine agonist and chemotherapeutic agents
Psychogenic	Anorexia, anxiety, stress, hysteria, schizophrenia

MANAGEMENT

Acute hiccups may be terminated by physical manoeuvres.

In contrast, there is insufficient evidence to guide the treatment of persistent or intractable hiccups with either pharmacological or non-pharmacological interventions.

Treatment is guided by the nature of the underlying cause.

Non-Pharmacological

- Physical manoeuvres
  - Interruption of the respiratory cycle
    (eg, holding breath, Valsalva manoeuvre or rebreathing into a paper bag — causing hypercapnia)
  - Irritation of the nasopharynx
    (eg, drinking water, pharyngeal stimulation)
  - Preventing diaphragmatic irritation
    (eg, leaning forward, pulling knees to chest)
- Acupuncture
- Hypnotherapy

Pharmacological

- Correct the underlying precipitant, particularly if the patient's prognosis allows time for the benefit to be appreciated:
  - Treat sepsis
  - Correct metabolic abnormalities
  - Stop drugs that may precipitate hiccups
- Manage gastric reflux (most common cause) and distension:
  - Omeprazole 10–40 mg BD
  - Domperidone 5–10 mg TDS

- — Metoclopramide 5–20 mg TDS
- Other drugs:
  - — Chlorpromazine 12.5–50 mg TDS-QDS (this is the only FDA approved drug for hiccups but it can cause sedation)
  - — Haloperidol 0.5–1 mg TDS
  - — Gabapentin 100–300 mg TDS
  - — Clonazepam 0.5–1 mg BD
  - — Baclofen 5–10 mg TDS
  - — SC Midazolam 10–60 mg/24 hours (may be useful in cases of terminal illness)

PRACTICAL TIPS

1. If no cause is found, then empirical treatment to suppress GERD provides relief in some individuals.
2. Metoclopramide is recommended as the first choice for peripheral causes. Domperidone may be safer for long term treatment.
3. Baclofen is the first line therapy for central causes of persistent hiccups. Gabapentin may also be safe and effective in long-term management of this condition.
4. Clinical experience also supports the use of chlorpromazine for acute but not long-term management.
5. Peripheral anaesthetic blocks to nerves involved in the putative hiccup 'reflex arc', surgical disruption or stimulation of vagal afferents or phrenic efferent nerves can be considered as final resort.

REFERENCES

1. Calsina-Berna A, et al. Treatment of chronic hiccups in cancer patients: A systematic review. *J Palliat Med*. 2012;15(10):1142–50.
2. Moretto EN, *et al*. Interventions for treating persistent and intractable hiccups in adults. *Cochrane Database of Syst Rev*. 2013;2013(1):CD008768.
3. Steger, M, *et al*. Systematic review: The pathogenesis and pharmacological treatment of hiccups. *Aliment Pharmacol Ther*. 2015;42:1037–1050.
4. Jeon YS, *et al*. Management of hiccups in palliative care patients. *BMJ Support Palliat Care*. 2018;8:1–6.

MALIGNANT ASCITES

Ang Ching Ching, Allyn Hum and Heng Xiaowei

INTRODUCTION

Ascites is a pathological condition where there is an excessive accumulation of fluid in the peritoneal cavity.

The amount of fluid available for normal physiological function is reduced as ascites has trapped the body fluid in a 'third space' where it cannot escape.

Malignant ascites is often a manifestation of end-stage advanced cancer and is associated with a poor prognosis.

Clinical Manifestations of Ascites

Patients commonly complain of abdominal distension, a 'stretching', 'pulling' pain, early satiety and dyspnoea (diaphragmatic splinting).

CAUSES

Malignant ascites may be seen with ovarian, breast, colorectal, lung, pancreatic, and liver cancers.

Malignant disease can contribute to ascites through the following mechanisms:

- Peritoneal carcinomatosis (53%)
- Massive liver metastasis causing portal hypertension (13%)

- Peritoneal carcinomatosis plus massive liver metastasis (13%)
- Hepatocellular carcinoma plus cirrhosis (13%)
- Chylous ascites due to malignancy, usually lymphoma (7%)
- Budd-Chiari syndrome due to malignancy occluding the hepatic veins (Rare)

INVESTIGATIONS

Peritoneal fluid should be evaluated for portal hypertension, the presence of malignant cells and to exclude peritonitis.
- Cell count and differential count
  — Bacterial peritonitis may be present if WBCs ≥250 cells/mm^3
- Serum-Ascites Albumin Gradient (SAAG)
  — SAAG ≥11 g/L suggests portal hypertension (transudative) with 97% accuracy, and patients may respond to diuretics
- Gram stain and culture
- Cytology

MANAGEMENT

Non-Pharmacological

- Abdominal paracentesis is the mainstay of treatment
  — Symptom relief in 90% of patients, and frequency of drainage guided by patient's symptoms
- Indwelling tunnelled catheters (PleurX) may facilitate paracentesis for symptomatic recurrent malignant ascites
  — Advantages: Reduces hospitalisations for drainage
  — Limitations: Drain site leakage, infections (drain site, loculated ascites, peritonitis), hypotension, electrolyte imbalances

Pharmacological

- If SAAG ≥11 g/L (portal hypertension present), Frusemide combined with Spironolactone in the ratio of 2 : 5 may be useful if blood pressure permits

- PO Morphine Sulphate syrup 2.5 mg 4–6 hourly
  - Opioids may relieve distressing symptoms from malignant ascites
  - However, Morphine Sulphate is metabolised in the liver and excreted by the kidneys
    In patients with renal (CrCl <30 mL/min) and/or hepatic impairment (AST and/or ALT ≥3 times upper normal limit), consider either dose reduction by 25–50%, extending dose interval to 8 hourly, or to switch to fentanyl

PRACTICAL TIPS

1. It is generally safe to remove 2–4 L of peritoneal fluid daily (blood pressure permitting).
2. There is no proven benefit of giving blood products to reverse coagulopathy before, or concomitant plasma expanders (IV Albumin, Normal Saline) during paracentesis.

REFERENCES

1. Becker G, Galandi D, Blum HE. Malignant ascites: Systemic review and guideline for treatment. *Eur J Cancer.* 2006;42:589.
2. Burleigh K, Mehta Z, Ellison N. Tunneled indwelling catheters for malignant ascites #308. *J Palliat Med.* 2016;19:671.
3. Gines P, Cardenas A. Management of cirrhosis and ascites. *New Engl J Med.* 2004;350(16):1646–1654.
4. Narayanan G, Pezeshkmehr A, Venkat S, *et al.* Safety and efficacy of the PleurX catheter for the treatment of malignant ascites. *J Palliat Med.* 2014;17:906.
5. Parsons SL, Watson SA. Malignant ascites. *Br J Surg.* 1996;83:6–14.
6. Rosenberg SM. Palliation of malignant ascites. *Gastroenterol Clin North Am.* 2006;35:189–199.
7. Wong BC, Cake L, Kachuik L, Amjadi K. Indwelling peritoneal catheters for managing malignancy-associated ascites. *J Palliat Care.* 2015;31:243.

NAUSEA AND VOMITING

Ong Wah Ying and Heng Xiaowei

INTRODUCTION

Nausea is an unpleasant feeling of the need to vomit, often accompanied by autonomic symptoms whilst vomiting is the forceful expulsion of gastric contents through the mouth. This differs from regurgitation, which is the reflux of oesophageal contents to the hypopharynx.

CAUSES

Common causes include:

Neurological	• Migraine
	• Space-occupying lesions (malignancy, abscess)
	• Cerebrovascular (haemorrhage, infarction)
Psychological	• Anxiety, pain and anticipatory nausea
Gastrointestinal	• Obstruction ('squashed stomach syndrome', gastric outlet obstruction, small/large bowel obstruction, constipation)
	• Gastroparesis
	• Gastric irritation (infections, bleeding)
Metabolic	• Renal failure, hypercalcemia
Iatrogenic	• Opioids, antibiotics and NSAIDs
	• Chemotherapy-induced
	• Radiotherapy-induced

CHARACTERISTICS OF ANTI-EMETICS

There are many neurotransmitter receptors involved in nausea and vomiting. The vomiting centre is located in the brainstem and it coordinates the processes involved in vomiting. It may be activated by stimuli from the chemoreceptor trigger zone (CTZ), the gastrointestinal tract, the vestibular apparatus, and the cerebral cortex.

Consider the route of administration when ordering anti-emetics (These medications are available locally).

Receptors	Anti-Emetics Class	Examples
Vomiting Centre (VC)		
• Acetylcholine (ACh)	• Anticholinergic	• Hyoscine hydrobromide (Scopolamine)
• Serotonin (5-HT$_2$)	• 5-HT$_2$ antagonist	• Olanzapine
• Histaminergic (H1)	• Antihistaminergic (H1)	• Olanzapine
Chemoreceptor Trigger Zone (CTZ)		
• Dopamine (D$_2$)	• Antidopaminergic	• Haloperidol • Olanzapine • Metoclopramide • Domperidone • Prochlorperazine (Stemetil)
• Serotonin (5-HT$_3$)	• 5-HT$_3$ antagonist	• Ondansetron • Palonosetron • Metoclopramide
• Neurokinin (NK$_1$)	• NK$_1$ antagonist	• Aprepitant (Specialist advice required)
GI Tract		• Metoclopramide
• Serotonin (5-HT$_3$)	• 5-HT$_3$ antagonist	• Ondansetron • Metoclopramide

(Continued)

(*Continued*)

Receptors	Anti-Emetics Class	Examples
• Serotonin (5-HT$_4$) • Dopamine (D$_2$)	• 5-HT$_4$ antagonist • Antidopaminergic	• Metoclopramide • Haloperidol • Olanzapine • Metoclopramide • Domperidone
• Mechanoreceptors & chemoreceptors	• Anti-secretory agents to decrease intra-luminal pressure	• Octreotide • Hyoscine butylbromide (Buscopan) • Ranitidine • Famotidine
Vestibular Apparatus		
• Histaminergic (H$_1$)	• Antihistaminergic	• Prochlorperazine (Stemetil)
• Acetylcholine (ACh)	• Anticholinergic	• Hyoscine hydrobromide (Scopolamine)

PHARMACOLOGICAL MANAGEMENT

Chemoreceptor Trigger Zone (CTZ)

- Chemotherapy-induced nausea and vomiting: 4-drug combination of an NK$_1$ antagonist, 5-HT3 antagonist, Dexamethasone, and Olanzapine for high-emetic-risk chemotherapy
- Opioid-induced nausea: PO/IV/SC Metoclopramide 10 mg TDS (up to 1 mg/kg) or PO/SC Haloperidol 0.5–1.5 mg TDS

Cerebral Cortex

- Raised intracranial pressure from brain metastasis: PO/IV/SC Dexamethasone 8–24 mg/24 hr with proton-pump inhibitor cover

Gastrointestinal Tract

- Nasogastric tube decompression if persistently vomiting

- Partial/Incomplete obstruction:
  i) For vomiting:
  IV/SC Metoclopramide 10 mg TDS. If persistent, to consider IV/SC Metoclopramide infusion up to 1 mg/kg/day.

  ii) For adjunct to reduce gastric secretions:
  Add IV/SC Ranitidine 50–200 mg/24 hr. (CrCl < 50 mL/min, renal adjustment dose is 50 mg/24 hr).
  Alternatively, IV/SC Famotidine 40 mg/24 hr. (CrCl < 50 mL/min, renal adjustment dose is 20 mg/24hr).

  iii) For reduction of gut edema:
  Consider a 3–5 days trial of IV/SC Dexamethasone 8–12 mg/24 hr with proton-pump inhibitor cover (if no contraindications).

- Complete obstruction:
  i) For vomiting:
  IV/SC Haloperidol 5 mg/24 hr infusion or Sublingual Olanzapine 2.5 mg OD-BD for nausea.

  ii) For adjunct to reduce gastric secretions:
  Add IV/SC Ranitidine 50–200 mg/24 hr. (CrCl < 50 mL/min, renal adjustment dose is 50 mg/24 hr).
  Alternatively, IV/SC Famotidine 40 mg/24 hr. (CrCl < 50 mL/min, renal adjustment dose is 20 mg/24hr).

  iii) For reduction of gut secretions:
  IV/SC Hyoscine Butylbromide (Buscopan) 60–120 mg/24 hr for reduction of GI secretions.
  IV/SC Octreotide 100 mcg 8 hourly or as continuous IV/SC infusion 300mcg-900mcg /24hr.

  iv) For reduction of gut edema:
  Consider a 3–5 days trial of IV/SC Dexamethasone 8–12 mg/24 hr with proton-pump inhibitor cover (if no contraindications).

Vestibular

- Labyrinthitis: PO Prochlorperazine (Stemetil) 5–10 mg TDS

PRACTICAL TIPS

1. Metoclopramide and Domperidone are prokinetic agents.
   - **DO NOT USE** in impending or complete intestinal obstruction due to the risk of perforation.
2. Hyoscine Butylbromide (Buscopan) reduces colic and secretions in the GI tract which can contribute to a patient's nausea. It may, however, worsen ileus.
3. Olanzapine acts on **multiple sites** (antidopaminergic, anticholinergic, antihistaminergic and 5-HT$_3$ antagonist) and is an effective anti-emetic that can be given sublingually.

REFERENCES

1. Clark K, Lam L, Currow D. Reducing gastric secretions — A role for histamine 2 antagonists or proton pump inhibitors in malignant bowel obstruction?. *Support Care Cancer.* 2009;17(12):1463–1468.
2. Crawford G, Gastrointestinal symptoms. In: *Therapeutic Guidelines Palliative Care*, Version 2; 2005, pp. 209–216.
3. Hesketh PJ, Kris MG, Basch E, *et al*. Antiemetics: American Society of Clinical Oncology guideline update. *J Clin Oncol.* 2020;38(24):2782–2797.
4. Singh P, Yoon SS, Kuo B. Nausea: A review of pathophysiology and therapeutics. *Therap Adv Gastroenterol.* 2016;9:98.
5. Watson M, Lucas C, Hoy A, Back I. Symptom management; Gastrointestinal symptoms. In: Chap. 6, *Oxford Handbook of Palliative Care*; 2005, pp. 246–253.
6. Woodruff R. Gastrointestinal symptoms. In: *Palliative Medicine*, 4th ed. 2004; pp. 223–233.

ORAL THRUSH

Chia Siew Chin

INTRODUCTION

Oral candidiasis is not common in the general population, but may be common in immunocompromised patients. In the United States, the prevalence has been estimated to be nearly 20% in cancer patients.

Patients may experience altered taste sensations and odynophagia.

Candida albicans is the most common organism involved. Other species like *Candida krusei* have appeared in immuno-compromised persons. *Candida glabrata* is an emerging cause in patients with head and neck cancer undergoing radiotherapy.

Oral candidiasis may manifest in different forms. The pseudomembranous form is most commonly seen with white plaques seen on an erythematous base. Others are the atrophic form with a diffuse erythema without white plaques, the hyperplastic form with leukoplakia and angular cheilitis.

CAUSES

- Xerostomia: post-radiotherapy or chemotherapy for head and neck cancers or drug-induced xerostomia
- Poor oral hygiene: including poorly cleaned dentures
- Smoking: significantly increases the carriage of *Candida*
- Corticosteroids: topical, systemic or inhaled

- Diabetes: due to increased glucose content in the saliva
- Prolonged antibiotics or immuno-modulating drugs: due to disruption of normal oral flora

MANAGEMENT

Pharmacological

Oral Candidiasis

Treatment can be divided into topical or oral/intravenous systemic treatment.

Topical

For mild disease:
- Nystatin solution/lozenges (100,000 u/ml) 5 ml QDS
  — to be swished and swallowed for a duration of 7–14 days
- Gentian violet topical solution/Clotrimazole topical solutions/ lozenges
  — can be used in the rare case when there is resistance to Nystatin (rare)

Oral Antifungals

For moderate to severe disease or refractory to topical treatment:
- Fluconazole at a dosage of 100–200 mg (3 mg/kg) OM for 7–14 days
- Itraconazole solution 200 mg daily (80% with infection refractory to Fluconazole will respond to Itraconazole solution) or Posaconazole 400 mg BD for 3 days followed by 400 mg OM for up to 28 days

Oesophageal Candidiasis

Requires systemic and not topical antifungals:
- Fluconazole 200–400 mg (3–6 mg/kg) daily for 14–21 days
- IV Fluconazole 400 mg/day (6 mg/kg) or Amphotericin B 0.3–0.7 mg/kg daily

— For Fluconazole-refractory disease, Itraconazole, Posaconazole or Voriconazole oral or intravenous solutions can be used at similar doses as above but for a longer duration of 14–21 days
— An antifungal trial should be initiated before endoscopic examination is done (Consult the infectious disease physician before starting)

PRACTICAL TIPS

1. Oral *candidiasis* should be treated to improve symptoms and prevent oesophageal candidiasis.
2. Take out dentures between meals.
3. Reduce the dose and duration of steroids.
4. Limit the duration of broad-spectrum antibiotics.
5. A toothette may be used to apply the topical antifungal solution if the patient cannot swish and swallow the solution.

REFERENCES

1. Davies N, Brailsford SR. Oral candidiasis in community-based patients with advanced cancer. *J Pain Symptom Manage*. 2008;35(5):508–514.
2. Pappas P, Kauffman CA. Clinical practice guidelines for the management of candidiasis: 2009 update by the infectious diseases society of America. *Clin Infect Dis*. 2009;48(5):503–535.

PRURITUS

Allyn Hum and Heng Xiaowei

INTRODUCTION

Itching, when intractable, is disabling and can add to a patient's distress towards the end of life.

The sensation arises when free nerve endings found superficially in the skin are stimulated by a variety of chemicals, such as histamine, serotonin, prostaglandins, kinins, proteases and endothelin.

CAUSES OF PRURITIS

- Dermatological
  - Xerosis
  - Eczema
  - Psoriasis
- Medical conditions
  - Metabolic: Hyperparathyroidism, hypo/hyperthyroidism
  - Haematological: Polycythaemia, iron deficiency anaemia
  - Hepatic failure
  - Renal failure
  - Lymphoproliferative/solid tumours (paraneoplastic)
- Infections
  - Scabies
  - Lice
  - *Candida*

- Drug induced
  - Morphine and related opioids
- Allergy
  - Urticaria
  - Contact dermatitis
- Psychogenic

MANAGEMENT

Where possible, management should be targeted towards rectifying the underlying cause, e.g. palliative cytoreductive therapy for malignancy.

TREATMENT MODALITIES

General Skin Care

- Regular use of emollients, which add hydration to soothe and repair skin
  - Occlusives have a thick and heavy consistency to form a physical barrier to prevent water loss from the skin's surface e.g. paraffin
  - Humectants extract water molecules from the air and into the skin e.g. urea cream, ceramides
- Non-soap cleansers e.g. emulsifying ointment
- Cool, airy environment e.g. light-weight clothing
- Avoid hot baths

End-Stage Renal Failure

- Topical emollients, e.g. Dermaveen/Aveeno (colloidal oatmeal), Suu Balm (menthol)
  - Oatmeal or menthol-based emollient creams are usually more effective in pruritis of renal failure, reducing itching and redness
- Antihistamines (Chlorpheniramine 4 mg TDS/Hydroxyzine 10–25 mg TDS)
- Antidepressants
  - SSRI (Sertraline 25–50 mg OD/Paroxetine 10–40 mg OM)

— SNRI (Mirtazapine 7.5–15 mg ON)
— TCA (Doxepin 10–30 mg ON for intractable cases)
- Anticonvulsants (Gabapentin 100 ON-TDS)
- 5-HT3 antagonists (Ondansetron 4–8 mg TDS)
- Phototherapy (UVB light therapy, UVA therapy with psoralen)

Uremic Pruritis

- sc Erythropoietin 36 IU/kg 3x weekly

Hepatic Cholestasis

- Cholestyramine 4 g BD-TDS
- Rifampicin 10 mg/kg OM
- UVB light therapy

Haematological Causes

- Iron Replacement (till Ferritin levels are normal)
- Aspirin (for Polycythaemia rubra vera)
- UVB light therapy
- UVA therapy with psoralen

PRACTICAL TIPS

1. In many cases, a combination of several drugs may be required to effectively control the patient's pruritus.
2. Opioid-induced pruritus is often transient due to an initial reaction caused by histamine release. It should resolve within a few hours or days.

REFERENCES

1. Ko MJ, Yang JY, Wu HY, *et al*. Narrowband ultraviolet B phototherapy for patients with refractory uraemic pruritis: a randomized controlled trial. *Bri J Dermatol*. 2011;165:633.

2.   Kouwenhoven TA, van de Kerkhof PCM, Kamsteeg M. Use of oral antidepressants in patients with chronic pruritis: A systematic review. *J Am Acad Dermatol.* 2017;77:1068.

3.   Krajnik M, Zylicz Z. Understanding pruritus in systemic disease. *J Pain Symptom Manage.* 2001;21:151–168.

4.   Matsuda KM, Sharma D, Schonfeld AR, Kwatra SG. Gabapentin and pregabalin for the treatment of chronic pruritus. *J Am Acad Dermatol.* 2016;75:619.

5.   Yosipovitch G, Bernhard JD. Clinical practice. Chronic pruritis. *New Engl J Med.* 2013;368:1625.

6.   Zylicz Z, Krajnik M. Managing severe pruritus in cancer patients. *Eur J Palliat Care.* 2007;14:93–95.

7.   De Marchi S, Cecchin E, Villalta D, Sepiacci G, Santini G, Bartoli E. Relief of pruritus and decreases in plasma histamine concentrations during erythropoietin therapy in patients with uremia. *N Engl J Med.* 1992 Apr 9;326(15):969–974.

SECTION 3: END ORGAN DISEASE

END-STAGE HEART FAILURE

Aw Chia Hui

INTRODUCTION

The symptom burden and psychosocial needs of patients with heart failure (HF) is comparable to that in advanced cancer. Palliative care improves symptom control, quality of life (QOL), psycho-spiritual well-being and reduces HF-related readmissions in patients with HF.

CLASSIFICATION OF HF

NYHA Functional Classification		ACC/AHA Stages of HF	
I	No limitation of physical activity. Ordinary physical activity does not cause symptoms of HF.	A	At high risk for HF but without structural heart disease or symptoms of HF.
II	Slight limitation of physical activity. Comfortable at rest, but ordinary physical activity results in symptoms of HF.	B	Structural heart disease but without signs or symptoms of HF.
III	Marked limitation of physical activity. Comfortable at rest, but less than ordinary physical activity results in symptoms of HF.	C	Structural heart disease with prior or current symptoms of HF.

(Continued)

(Continued)

NYHA Functional Classification	ACC/AHA Stages of HF
IV Unable to carry on any physical activity without symptoms of HF, or symptoms of HF at rest.	D Refractory HF requiring specialised interventions.

Abbreviations: NYHA = New York Heart Association, ACC/AHA = American College of Cardiology/American Heart Association.

FEATURES OF ADVANCED HF

- NYHA Class III/IV or ACC/AHA Stage D
- Intolerance to neurohormonal therapy (ACE-I, Beta-blockers) due to persistent hypotension or worsening renal function
- Increasingly refractory to diuretics with high doses needed to maintain fluid status (usually daily frusemide equivalent dose >160 mg/day or need for supplemental Metolazone therapy)
- Progressive hyponatremia (Na<133 mmol/L)
- Anaemia (Hb<13 g/dL in men and <12 g/dL in women)
- Progressive deterioration in renal or liver function
- Repeated heart-failure related admissions (>2 in a year)
- Unintentional weight loss (cardiac cachexia)
- Frequent ICD shocks

DISEASE TRAJECTORY IN HF

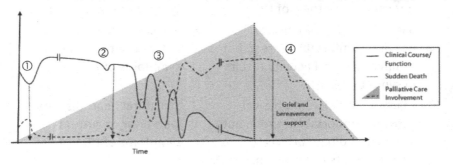

Fig. 1: Depiction of the disease trajectory and role of palliative care in patients with HF. Palliative care may be involved at ① Initial diagnosis, ② During episodes of acute deterioration, as patients progress into ③ Advanced HF and for ④ Bereavement support (which may begin at any point in the trajectory if sudden death occurs)

PROGNOSTICATION IN HF

Prognostication is often challenging due to the unpredictable disease trajectory with high incidence (up to 50%) of sudden death.

In general, 1-year mortality for patients with NYHA Class IV is around 30–40%. Prognostic models such as the Seattle HF model and EFFECT model predict all-cause mortality of 1 year or less, while the ADHERE model predicts the risk of in-hospital mortality. However, these models are not easily applicable by the bedside. It must be emphasised that consideration of patient care needs must take precedence over prognostic uncertainties when considering referral to palliative or hospice services.

SYMPTOM MANAGEMENT IN ADVANCED HF

There are limited high-quality studies on symptom management in advanced HF. Much of the following recommendations are postulated from studies in patients with COPD or advanced cancer.

Dyspnoea

Dyspnoea is common and reversible causes such as fluid overload, anemia, or underlying comorbidities such as COPD or renal failure should be evaluated and managed appropriately.

Non-pharmacological management includes the use of a fan directed to the face, ambulatory oxygen in patients hypoxemic at rest/on exertion (PaO_2<55 mmHg or SaO_2<92%) and cardiac rehabilitation.

While diuretics and vasodilatory agents are usually first-line in the pharmacological management of dyspnoea in HF, their use is often limited by hypotension or renal impairment. Opioids such as oral morphine 2.5 mg 4–6 hourly can be started for mild to moderate dyspnoea. In patients with liver or renal impairment, a longer dosing interval may be required. In patients with moderate to severe dyspnoea, an opioid infusion may be started and titrated to effect.

Anxiety frequently accompanies dyspnoea and low doses of benzodiazepines such as PO alprazolam 0.25–0.5 mg TDS PRN or PO lorazepam 0.5–1 mg ON PRN may be helpful.

Oedema

Fluid overload and hypoalbuminemia from cardiac cachexia can cause distressing lower limb oedema or anasarca. Diuretics remain the mainstay of treatment. Oral bumetanide has greater bioavailability compared to frusemide and is a useful alternative (Bumetanide : Frusemide potency = 1 mg : 40 mg). Supplemental metolazone 2.5–20 mg can also be added to loop diuretics. Renal function should be monitored during the use of diuretics.

Fatigue

Up to 85% of patients with advanced HF report feeling fatigued but this is often under-recognised. Reversible causes such as anaemia, electrolyte derangements, sleep disturbances and medication use (e.g., anticholinergics) should be evaluated and treated. Intravenous iron therapy in iron-deficient patients (Fe<100 or Fe Sat<20%) also improves fatigue, physical function and QOL, independent of the presence of anaemia.

Pain

Pain affects up to 75% of patients with advanced HF in the last six months of life. Common causes include (non-exhaustive):

- Cardiac-related such as angina
- Comorbidities such as ischemic pain from peripheral vascular disease, neuropathic pain from diabetic peripheral neuropathy and musculoskeletal pain from inactivity.
- Acute gout flares precipitated by the use of diuretics are also common.

The underlying precipitant of pain should be treated, such as the use of steroids or colchicine in acute gout flare. Nitrates remain first-line in the treatment of angina and opioids may be considered for those who suffer persistent angina or in whom nitrates are contraindicated. Analgesic use should be titrated according to the WHO pain ladder, with the addition of pain adjuvants if neuropathic pain is present.

Note that the use of NSAIDs or COX-2 inhibitors is contraindicated in HF.

Cardiac Cachexia

Cardiac cachexia is defined as the unintentional loss of >5% oedema-free body weight in the last 12 months and at least three of the following: decreased muscle strength, fatigue, anorexia, low fat-free muscle mass and abnormal biochemistry (raised CRP, IL-6, Hb<12 g/dL or alb<32 g/L).

Management is multimodal, targeted at optimising nutritional intake (nutritional supplements), controlling factors that may impair oral intake (e.g. good oral care and treatment of oral thrush) and exercise training. A trial of Renin-Aldosterone-Angiotensin-system (RAAS) blockade (e.g. Enalapril) or beta-blockers may be offered.

Anxiety/Depression

HF patients may also suffer from psychological symptoms like anxiety and depression (refer to respective chapters).

'TRIGGERS' FOR REFERRAL TO PALLIATIVE CARE IN ADVANCED HF

Patients with the following needs may benefit from referral to palliative care:

- Ongoing symptoms of HF with poor QOL despite optimal pharmacological and non-pharmacological therapies
- Advanced HF with progressive physical/cognitive decline or cardiac cachexia, deemed unsuitable for advanced cardiac therapies
- Concomitant life-limiting condition (advanced cancer, advanced dementia, other end-organ impairment, frailty)
- The physician would not be surprised if the patient died within the next 12 months

- Need for psychoemotional/spiritual support to patient or family (e.g. risk for complicated grief)
- Complex communications with patient or family (e.g. disagreement in goals of care between patient, family or medical team, withdrawal of life-sustaining treatment)
- Care coordination (e.g. Need for home hospice support, palliative home inotropic therapy or inpatient hospice)

ADVANCED THERAPIES AND DEVICE MANAGEMENT AT THE END OF LIFE

Inotropic Support

Inotropic support may be intermittent or continuous. Levosimendan is a calcium sensitiser that may be administered by HF specialists at intervals (up to months) for its inotropic effect.

Continuous home inotropic support, when used as long-term therapy for palliation of symptoms in advanced HF, should be initiated only in patients with adequate social support due to the complex logistics involved. Advance care planning, specifically addressing the end-points and limitations of inotropic support should be discussed *before* initiation. Home hospice teams, together with the HF team, may continue to support these patients in the community.

	Purpose	Outcome	Deactivation at EOL
PPM	Maintain Rhythm (Bradyarrhythmia)	Improve symptoms	No
ICD	Break tachyarrhythmia Most have PPM function	Prevent death	Yes (Defibrillator part only, do not deactivate PPM function)
CRT(D)	Synchronise/Pace ventricles	Improve symptoms +/− prevent death	Defibrillator part only

Abbreviation: PPM = Permanent pacemaker, ICD = implantable cardioverter-defibrillator CRT(D) = Cardiac Resynchronization Therapy Defibrillator.

Device Management

Deactivation of devices such as ICD should be discussed when:

- The patient expresses wish for deactivation
- Prognosis approaches days to weeks or death is imminent
- Do-Not-Resuscitate order initiated

Deactivation of devices can be psychologically distressing for patients and their families who may perceive that physicians are giving up hope or even attempting to hasten death. Discussions must be sensitively carried out and shared-decision making employed.

ADVANCE CARE PLANNING

Can be introduced and reviewed at diagnosis of HF, during acute exacerbations/hospitalisations, before initiation of advanced therapies such as inotropic support or device implantation, a decline in health or functional status, or as patients approach the terminal phase.

PRACTICAL TIPS

1. Use a combination of trigger criteria and the surprise question to identify patients who may benefit from the involvement of the palliative care team.
2. As part of symptom management, some cardiac medications such as diuretics, beta-blockers and nitrates may be continued until the last few weeks of life (unless contraindicated).
3. When possible, advance care planning and goals of care discussion should be initiated with patients and their family.

REFERENCES

1. Bekelman DB, Rumsfeld JS, Havranek EP, *et al*. Symptom burden, depression, and spiritual well-being: A comparison of HF and advanced cancer patients. *J Gen Intern Med*. May 2009;24(5):592–598. doi:10.1007/s11606-009-0931-y

2.   Rogers JG, Patel CB, Mentz RJ, *et al.* Palliative care in HF: The PAL-HF Randomized, Controlled Clinical Trial. *J Am Coll Cardiol.* Jul 18 2017;70(3): 331–341. doi:10.1016/j.jacc.2017.05.030
3.   Yancy CW, Jessup M, Bozkurt B, *et al.* 2013 ACCF/AHA guideline for the management of HF: A report of the American College of Cardiology Foundation/ American Heart Association Task Force on Practice Guidelines. *J Am Coll Cardiol.* Oct 15 2013;62(16):e147–239. doi:10.1016/j.jacc.2013.05.019
4.   Cleland JG, Chattopadhyay S, Khand A, Houghton T, Kaye GC. Prevalence and incidence of arrhythmias and sudden death in HF. *Heart Fail Rev.* Jul 2002; 7(3):229–242. doi:10.1023/a:1020024122726
5.   Zhou X, Xu W, Xu Y, Qian Z. Iron supplementation improves cardiovascular outcomes in patients with HF. *Am J Med.* Aug 2019;132(8):955–963. doi:10.1016/j.amjmed.2019.02.018

END-STAGE RENAL FAILURE

Jennifer Guan

INTRODUCTION

In Singapore, an average of 5 people are diagnosed with end stage renal disease every day, with the majority of them above the age of 60. These patients may choose to undergo kidney transplantation or other means of renal replacement therapy such as hemodialysis or peritoneal dialysis. There are also patients who are conservatively managed.

CLASSIFICATION OF END STAGE RENAL FAILURE

End stage renal disease (ESRD) is classified by the Kidney Disease: Improving Global Outcomes (KDIGO) guidelines as Stage 5 Chronic Kidney Disease (CKD) with an estimated glomerular filtration rate $</= 15$ ml/min per 1.73 m^2 or those requiring renal replacement therapy

PROGNOSTICATION IN END STAGE RENAL FAILURE

The majority of prognostication tools or predictive models are developed and validated in dialysis patients. Age is a major effect modifier in chronic kidney disease. Although dialysis for patients $>/= 70$ years does show a survival benefit, it is significantly diminished in patients who are older ($>/= 80$ years old) with more co-morbidities. There are various tools used

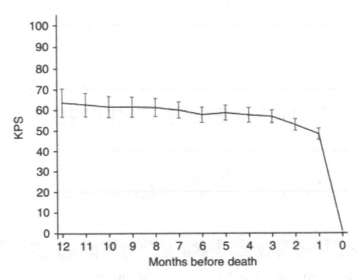

Fig. 1:   Trajectory of mean Karnofsky Performance Scale (KPS) scores over the last year of life for those who died with ESRD. Adapted from Murtagh *et al.*

to predict survival in ESRD patients such as the modified Charlson Co-morbidity Score, the Surprise Question and Dialysis initiation Risk Score.

For patients who are conservatively managed, the functional status is maintained until late in the course of illness, with rapid decline in the final weeks before death. This is also accompanied by a marked increase in their symptom burden in the last 1–2 months of life.

SYMPTOM MANAGEMENT

Patients with ESRD have a similar symptom burden whether they are on renal replacement therapy or not. These symptoms have contributing sources including renal failure, existing co-morbidities and dialysis therapies.

The initial approach in the management of these symptoms would be to evaluate and treat for reversible causes and modifiable factors. Please refer to the specific symptom chapters for further details on the management.

Table 1: Prevalence of Symptoms in Patients with ESRF Being Managed with and Without Dialysis.

Symptom	Symptom Prevalence (%)	
	Dialysis	Conservative
Fatigue/Tiredness	71	75
Pruritus	55	74
Constipation	53	
Anorexia	49	47
Pain	47	53
Sleep disturbances	44	42
Anxiety	38	
Dyspnea	35	61
Nausea	33	
Restless Legs	30	48
Depression	27	

Adapted from Brown *et al.*

Fatigue/Tiredness

Fatigue and tiredness are the most common symptoms in end stage renal disease patients and are often multifactorial. Whenever possible, treatment approach should be disease specific.

Non-Pharmacological Management

Apart from reassurance and patient education, it is prudent to assess the adequacy of dialysis with adjustments made in discussion with the primary renal physician.

Pharmacological Management

If it is due to the presence of anemia, it may be treated with blood transfusions, iron repletion therapy and/or adjusting the dose of erythropoietin. There is insufficient data on corticosteroids or psychostimulants in ESRD related fatigue.

Pain

Pain is another common symptom experienced by patients with CKD.

Causes include:

1. Primary kidney disease: polycystic kidney disease
2. Underlying comorbid conditions: diabetic neuropathy or peripheral vascular disease
3. Sequelae of CKD: calciphylaxis, bone pain from renal osteodystrophy
4. Dialysis related: complications from the arteriovenous fistula such as ischemic neuropathies, chronic infections, muscle cramps, peritonitis

Approximately 50% of patients report pain of moderate to severe intensity whether they are treated with dialysis or managed conservatively.

Pharmacological Management

For neuropathic pain, other classes of medication may need to be considered including tricyclic antidepressants or gabapentinoids. Based on the intensity of pain, we recommend following the WHO pain step ladder in analgesia administration, considering the renal clearance of the analgesic and its nature (i.e. whether the drug is removed during dialysis).

Dyspnea

Reversible causes should be evaluated and ruled out. Causes specific in ESRD to consider include fluid overload, anemia, cardiorenal complications and metabolic acidosis.

Pharmacological Management

Opioids are used for the management of dyspnea. However, many have active metabolites that can accumulate in patients with renal failure.

A lower dose/longer dosing interval may be required with careful titration.

Pharmacological management includes oral mist morphine 2.5 mg Q6 to 8 hourly for mild to moderate dyspnea. Alternatively, a fentanyl infusion may be initiated (Starting dose of SC Fentanyl at 10 mcg/hour for opioid naïve patients) and titrated to effect if the patient is unable to swallow or for the management of moderate to severe dyspnea.

As a significant population of these patients also experience anxiety and insomnia, the use of benzodiazepines such as alprazolam 0.25–0.5 mg TDS PRN and/or lorazepam 0.5 mg–1 mg ON PRN can be considered.

Uraemic Pruritus

The pathophysiology is multifactorial and poorly understood. Common causes include dry skin, inadequate dialysis, iron deficiency, secondary hyperparathyroidism and increased calcium/magnesium/phosphate deposition in the skin. Consider other causes of pruritus and manage accordingly.

Non-Pharmacological Management

Oat based topical emollients and avoidance of extremes of temperature.

Pharmacological Management

Gabapentin 100 mg after dialysis or every other day titrated to effect but not more than 300 mg daily may also help.

Restless Legs Syndrome

Associated with iron deficiency or hyperphosphatemia, it causes sleep disturbance, affecting quality of life. The international restless legs syndrome study group definition:

1. The desire to move the legs in association with unusual or uncomfortable sensations deep within the legs

2. Motor restlessness in an effort to remove these sensations
3. Symptoms become obvious or worse at rest and may be temporarily diminished by voluntary movement
4. Symptoms occur most frequently in the evening or early part of the night

Pharmacological Management

Gabapentin 100 mg once a day or after dialysis or a dopamine agonist such as ropinirole.

Seizures/Myoclonic Jerks

Uremic encephalopathy may lead to seizures and/or myoclonic jerks in ESRD patients. Other causes of seizures in these patients are similar to the general population and will also need to be assessed and ruled out.

Pharmacological Management

Benzodiazepines such as midazolam 1.5 mg–2 mg Q15 minutes may be initiated and titrated to effect.

IMPORTANT ISSUES: DIALYSIS WITHDRAWAL

Most patients who withdrew from dialysis survived a median of 7.4 days (range 0–40 days). Agitation, seizures and dyspnea are common terminal symptoms post withdrawal. The psychology of withdrawal for the patient and family may be emotionally fraught and requires careful and sensitive communication, coupled with the active pursuit of comfort and appropriate management of the terminal phase.

TRIGGERS FOR PALLIATIVE CARE REFERRALS

• Ongoing symptoms with poor QOL despite optimal pharmacological and non-pharmacological therapies in dialysis and non-dialysis patients.

- Medical condition precludes technical process of dialysis (patient unable to cooperate or recurrent hypotension during dialysis) or results in frequent hospitalisations and withdrawal of dialysis is being considered.
- Concomitant life-limiting condition (advanced cancer, irreversible or profound neurological impairment, other end-organ impairment, frailty).
- The clinician will not be surprised if patient demise occurs in the next 12 months or if there was rapid functional decline.
- Need for psycho-emotional/spiritual support to patient or family (e.g. risk for complicated grief).
- Complex communications with patient or family (e.g. disagreement in goals of care between patient, family or medical team, withdrawal of dialysis).
- Care coordination (e.g. Need for home hospice support, palliative home inotropic therapy or inpatient hospice).

PRACTICAL TIPS

1. Consider reversible causes for symptoms that develop in ESRD patients and treat accordingly.
2. Constant reassessment of symptoms should be done for these patients as they often change with time.
3. When and if possible, goals of care/advance care planning should be offered and discussed with the patient and family.

REFERENCES

1. KDIGO. Clinical Practice Guideline for the Evaluation and Management of Chronic Kidney Disease, 2010.
2. Advisor, SRR. *Singapore Renal Registry Annual Registry Report.* 1999–2014; 1999–2014: 2015: 1–13.
3. Murtagh FEM, Addington-Hall JM, Higginson IJ. End-stage renal disease: A new trajectory of functional decline in the last year of life. *J Am Geriatr. Soc.* 2011;59(2):304–308.

4. Brown MA, Crail SM. ANZSN. Renal supportive care guidelines 2013. The often difficult decision of which patients will benefit from Dialysis. *Nephrology*. 2013;18:401–454.
5. Davison SN. End-of-life care preferences and needs: Perceptions of patients with chronic kidney disease. *Clin J Am Soc Nephrol*. 2010;5(2):195–204.

END-STAGE LUNG DISEASE

Chiam Zi Yan

INTRODUCTION

Chronic Obstructive Pulmonary Disease (COPD) and Interstitial Lung Disease (ILD) are progressive life-limiting conditions. Palliative care involves close attention to the physical, emotional, spiritual, practical needs and goals of patients and of those who are close to them. It is recommended that palliative care be introduced alongside therapies aimed at reducing the risk of exacerbations and correcting the underlying pathophysiological abnormalities.

CLASSIFICATION OF COPD SEVERITY

Global Initiative of Chronic Obstructive Lung Disease

Classification of Severity of Airflow Limitation in COPD (Based on Post-Bronchodilator FEV1)		
GOLD 1	Mild	FEV1 ≥ 80% predicted
GOLD 2	Moderate	50% ≤ FEV1 < 80% predicted
GOLD 3	Severe	30% ≤ FEV1 < 50% predicted
GOLD 4	Very Severe	FEV1 < 30% predicted

Individualised Assessment of COPD

GOLD 4	C	D	≥2	
	High risk,	High risk,		Exacerbations per year
GOLD 3	less symptoms	more symptoms		
GOLD 2	A	B	0–1	
	Low risk,	Low risk,		
GOLD 1	less symptoms	more symptoms		
	mMRC* 0–1	mMRC* ≥2		
	CAT⁺ <10	CAT⁺ ≥10		

*mMRC (Modified Medical Research Council) Dyspnea Scale is a self-rating tool to measure degree of disability that breathlessness poses on scale of 0 (Dyspnea only with strenuous exercise) to 4 (Too dyspneic to leave house or when dressing).
⁺COPD Assessment Test (CAT) measures severity of cough, phlegm, chest tightness, breathlessness, activities, confidence leaving home despite lung condition, sleep, energy on scale of 0 to 5 (most severe).

CLASSIFICATION OF ILD

- **Idiopathic Interstitial Pneumonias (IIPs):** Idiopathic pulmonary fibrosis (IPF), idiopathic nonspecific interstitial pneumonia, unclassifiable IIPs
- **Autoimmune ILD:** Rheumatoid arthritis ILD, interstitial pneumonia with autoimmune features, systemic sclerosis ILD, Sjogren's syndrome ILD, systemic lupus erythematous ILD, polymyositis and dermatomyositis ILD, mixed connective tissue disease ILD
- **Hypersensitivity pneumonitis**
- **Sarcoidosis**
- **Other ILDs:** ILDs related to occupational exposures

PROGNOSTICATION IN COPD

- **Poor prognostic factors:** Recurrent admissions for COPD exacerbations, on long term oxygen therapy, presence of right heart failure, history of ICU admissions/non-invasive ventilation

- **BODE Index** for COPD Survival: BMI, FEV1% of predicted, 6 minute walk distance, mMRC dyspnea scale predicts 4 year survival

PROGNOSTICATION IN ILD

- IPF carries a poor prognosis with a median survival of 2 to 3 years from diagnosis
- **Poor prognostic factors:** Older age, more comorbidities, on long term oxygen therapy, presence of pulmonary hypertension, exertional desaturation, usual interstitial pneumonia pattern on CT scan, FVC decline of 10–15% predicted, acute exacerbations
- **ILD-Gender-Age-Physiology (ILD-GAP) index:** Predicts the risk of mortality at 1, 2 and 3 years for chronic ILD at different stages

SYMPTOMS MANAGEMENT

Symptom Burden in Chronic Lung Diseases

Physical	Psychological	Social	Functional
• Dyspnea	• Insomnia	• Social isolation	• Deconditioning
• Cough	• Anxiety		
• Dry mouth	• Irritability	• Financial concerns	
• Fatigue	• Depression		
• Pain	• Loss of hope		
• Constipation and prostatism			

MANAGEMENT OF DYSPNEA

Non-Pharmacological Management of Dyspnea

1. **Reassurance, support and education for patients and caregivers**
2. **Oxygen therapy**
   - Beneficial for relief of breathlessness and survival in patients with hypoxemia.
   - May also relieve breathlessness even in patients who are not hypoxemic but for careful control of supplemental oxygen in COPD patients with pre-existing type 2 respiratory failure.

3. **Pulmonary rehabilitation**
   - Reverse deconditioning, energy conservation techniques, breathing exercises (pursed lip breathing, controlled breathing), ADL training and mobility aids.
4. **Hand-held fan**
   - Reduction in dyspnea by activation of V2 and V3 branches of trigeminal nerve.
5. **Advance care planning**
6. **Multi-professional integrated breathlessness service**
   - Integrated palliative and respiratory care services help improve mastery of breathlessness.

Pharmacological Management of Dyspnea

1. **Disease specific treatment:** compliance to inhalers, inhaler technique, nicotine withdrawal.
2. **Symptoms based treatment:**
   - Systemic opioids
   Not associated with changes to arterial blood gases, respiratory suppression or survival.
   - Anxiolytics
   Overall, slight non-significant trend towards beneficial effect in COPD.
   PO alprazolam 0.125 mg to 0.25 mg PRN 8H for panic attacks.
   Sublingual lorazepam 0.5 mg to 1 mg bedtime PRN for insomnia.
   - Antidepressants
   Mirtazapine 7.5 mg to 15 mg ON: improvement in dyspnea scores seen in case series.

MANAGEMENT OF COUGH

Non-Pharmacological Management of Cough
- Lifestyle advice: Eat small meals and earlier in the day.

Pharmacological Management of Cough
- Medical therapies for cough are uniformly not effective in ILD/COPD.
- Treat any reversible causes such as infection.

- Other potential causes of cough, such as GERD, ACE-I use, and postnasal drip, should be identified and addressed.
- Simple linctus, codeine linctus or low dose opioids and neuromodulators such as gabapentin might be helpful in some and can be considered empirically.

Advanced Therapies

Non-Invasive Ventilation (NIV)	High-Flow Nasal Cannula (HFNC) Oxygen Delivery
COPD: • NIV in acute COPD exacerbations with type 2 respiratory failure improves mortality and reduces the need for endotracheal intubation. • Limited evidence with modest improvement in breathlessness compared with standard supplemental oxygen. ILD: NIV prevented endotracheal intubation in a minority of patients. Outcome of ILD patients requiring NIV is poor.	HFNC allows oxygen delivery from a fraction of inspired oxygen of 21% to 100% with an ability to generate up to 60 L/minute of flow. Compared with NIV, HFNC is better tolerated, with reduced interruptions for oxygen administration and greater freedom with eating and communication towards the end of life. But there is still a lack of evidence in reducing breathlessness in COPD and ILD.

TRIGGERS FOR PALLIATIVE CARE REFERRAL

- Resting dyspnea poorly responsive to bronchodilators
- Decreased functional capacity: eg predicted FEV1 < 30%, assistance with transfers, activity intolerance
- Repeated hospitalizations for exacerbations
- Right heart failure from Cor Pulmonale

- Unintentional weight loss of >10% body weight over the past 6 months
- Meets criteria for long term oxygen therapy

PRACTICAL TIPS

1. COPD and ILD are life-limiting progressive lung diseases that are associated with high symptom burden, functional incapacitation, unaddressed psycho-emotional needs, reduced quality of life, reduced survival and high tertiary care utilization.
2. Apart from chronic cough and exertional dyspnea, many of these patients also experience GERD, constipation, anxiety and insomnia.
3. Disease course is unpredictable and palliative care input must be individualized according to the needs of patients and caregivers.
4. A multidisciplinary approach and effective communication are crucial to addressing the needs of the patient and caregivers throughout the disease course.
5. Use of non-pharmacological treatment like hand-held fans has been proven to be beneficial.

REFERENCES

1. Halpin DMG, *et al.* Palliative care for people with COPD: Effective but underused. *Eur Respir J.* 2018;51:1702645.
2. Maddocks M, *et al.* Palliative care and management of troublesome symptoms for people with chronic obstructive pulmonary disease. *Lancet.* 2017;390:988–1002.
3. Uronis HE, Ekstrom MP, Currow DC, *et al.* Oxygen for relief of dyspnoea in people with chronic obstructive pulmonary disease who would not qualify for home oxygen: A systematic review and meta-analysis. *Thorax.* 2015; 70:492–494.
4. Higginson, *et al.* An integrated palliative and respiratory care service for patients with advanced disease and refractory breathlessness: A randomised controlled trial. *Lancet Respir Med.* 2014;2:979–987.
5. Kreuter, *et al.* Palliative care in interstitial lung disease: Living well. *Lancet Respir Med.* 2017;Dec;5(12):968–980.

END-STAGE LIVER DISEASE

Joanna Lau

INTRODUCTION

End-stage liver disease (ESLD) is a progressive, irreversible illness where inflammation of hepatic cells leads to fibrosis and disruption of liver function. Terms such as advanced liver disease, liver failure and decompensated cirrhosis are used synonymously. It is a major cause of morbidity and mortality worldwide, and even when liver transplantation is considered, many become too ill before a suitable donor is found. The symptom prevalence in this patient group mirrors that of patients with cancer or other advanced organ failure. The most frequently reported symptoms include pain, breathlessness, muscle cramps, sleep disturbance, depression and anxiety.

PROGNOSTICATION IN ESLD

The disease trajectory in ESLD is variable, but many patients will experience persistent deteriorating function interjected with episodes of acute illness requiring hospitalisations.

Prognosis is influenced by multiple factors, including:

- Aetiology of liver failure
- Degree of hepatic decompensation
- Degree and severity of complications e.g. variceal bleeding

- Deterioration in other major organs e.g. hepatorenal or hepatopulmonary syndrome
- Comorbid disease

The two commonly used models:

1.   **Child-Pugh classification**

Parameter	Points Assigned		
	1	**2**	**3**
Ascites	Absent	Slight	Moderate
Bilirubin	<34 μmol/l	34–51 μmol/l	>51 μmol/l
Albumin	35 g/L	28–35 g/L	<28 g/L
Prothrombin time (Seconds over control)	<4	4–6	>6
INR	<1.7	1.7–2.3	>2.3
Encephalopathy	None	Grade 1–2	Grade 3–4

West Haven criteria for grading hepatic encephalopathy:

Grade	Features
0	No abnormalities detected.
1	Unawareness (mild), euphoria or anxiety, shortened attention span, impairment of calculation ability, lethargy or apathy.
2	Disorientation to time, obvious personality change, inappropriate behaviour.
3	Somnolence to stupor, still responsive to stimuli, confusion, gross disorientation, bizarre behaviour.
4	Coma

Child-Pugh Class	Score	1-Year Survival (%)	2-year Survival (%)
A	5–6	100	85
B	7–9	80	60
C	10–15	45	35

2.   Model for End-Stage Liver Disease (MELD) score

MELD = $3.8*\log_e$(serum bilirubin [mg/dL]) + $11.2*\log_e$(INR) + $9.6*\log_e$ (serum creatinine [mg/dL]) + 6.4

MELD Score	3-Month Survival (%)	6-Month Survival (%)	1-Year Survival (%)
0–9	98	98	93
10–19	94	92	86
20–29	80	78	71
30–39	47	40	37

MANAGEMENT

Non-Pharmacological

- Dietary sodium restriction to less than 2 g/day.
- Abdominal paracentesis for symptomatic ascites.
- In cases of refractory ascites, indwelling peritoneal catheter or transjugular intrahepatic portosystemic shunting (TIPS) can be considered but requires careful patient selection.

Pharmacological

- Treat underlying cause where appropriate.
- Antibiotics for concomitant infection.
- Mist morphine 2.5 mg 6–8 hourly for pain or dyspnoea. If there is a need for higher opioid doses and toxicity is a concern in view of significant liver impairment, Fentanyl is a suitable alternative.
- IV albumin should be administered after large-volume paracentesis to prevent circulatory dysfunction. The recommendation is for 6–8 g of 25% albumin per litre of ascites drained.
- Combination of Frusemide 40 mg OM and Spironolactone 100 mg OM may be useful for patients with recurrent ascites, but to avoid use if hypotensive.

IMPORTANT ISSUES

1. The abrupt onset of ESLD symptoms coupled with hope for a life-saving transplant often delays discussions pertaining to goals of care and end-of-life issues.
2. There is growing recognition that palliative care input is beneficial in patients both awaiting transplantation and post-transplantation, as it improves communication and patient satisfaction.
3. There are concerns about opioid use as there is a higher prevalence of pre-existing substance abuse in the ESLD population and fears that opioids may worsen hepatic encephalopathy. However, conservative opioid use for symptom control is safe and there is no known association with alcohol recidivism.

TRIGGERS FOR PALLIATIVE CARE REFERRAL

Criteria for considering specialist palliative care referral:
- Child-Pugh class C
- MELD score ≥14
- Complications such as ascites, bleeding varices, or hepatic encephalopathy that are refractory to treatment
- Severe muscle wasting and cachexia
- Development of hepatorenal syndrome or renal failure
- Functional decline
- Spiritual or existential distress
- Anticipatory grief
- Goals of care disagreements
- Need for coordination of care between inpatient and community sites

PRACTICAL TIP

1. Early advance care planning is recommended especially when prognosis may be less than 1 year or liver transplantation is considered.

REFERENCES

1. Peng J, Hepgul N, Higginson I, Gao W. Symptom prevalence and quality of life of patients with end-stage liver disease: A systematic review and meta-analysis. *Palliat Med*. 2019;33(1):24–36.
2. Potosek J, Curry M, Buss M, Chittenden E. Integration of palliative care in end-stage liver disease and liver transplantation. *J Palliat Med*. 2014;17(11): 1271–1277.
3. Wijdicks EFM. Hepatic encephalopathy. *New Engl J Med*. 2016;375:1660–1670.
4. European Association for the Study of the Liver. EASL clinical practice guidelines on the management of ascites, spontaneous bacterial peritonitis, and hepatorenal syndrome in cirrhosis. *J Hepatol*. 2010;53(3):397–417.
5. Runyon BA. Practice Guidelines Committee, American Association for the Study of Liver Diseases (AASLD). Management of adult patients with ascites due to cirrhosis. *Hepatology*. 2004;39:841–856.
6. Cox-North P, Doorenbos A, Shannon SE, Scott J, Curtis JR. The transition to end-of-life care in end-stage liver disease. *J Hosp Palliat Nurs*. 2013;15(4): 209–215.
7. Esteban JPG, Rein L, Szabo A, Saeian K, Rhodes M, Marks S. Attitudes of liver and palliative care clinicians toward specialist palliative care consultation for patients with end-stage liver disease. *J Palliat Med*. 2019;22(7):804–813.

DEMENTIA AND FRAILTY

Goh Wen Yang

INTRODUCTION

- Dementia is a progressive, neurodegenerative disorder involving one or more cognitive domains (learning and memory, language, executive function, complex attention, perceptual-motor and social cognition), interfering with independence in daily living.
- Common causes of dementia include Alzheimer's disease, vascular dementia, frontotemporal dementia, Lewy body dementia and mixed dementia.
- Frailty is defined as reduced strength and physiologic malfunctioning that increases an individual's susceptibility to increased dependency, vulnerability and death.
- Frailty can be understood from a phenotypic perspective (Fried's criteria) and/or the cumulative deficit perspective (Rockwood's Frailty Index).

STAGING AND PROGNOSIS

- The Functional Assessment Staging test (FAST) and Clinical Frailty Scale (CFS) are used to stage dementia and frailty respectively.

FAST Stage	FAST Description	CFS	Prognosis
1 — Normal Ageing	No difficulty either subjectively or objectively	1 Very fit 2 Well	Rockwood and colleagues studied acutely ill adults aged ≥65 years presenting to the Emergency Department. Hazard ratio for 6 months mortality was 1.67 (95% CI: 1.48–1.89) per 1-grade increase in CFS.
2 — Possible Mild Cognitive Impairment	Subjective functional deficit	3 Managing well	
3 — Mild Cognitive Impairment	Objective functional deficit that interferes with a person's most complex tasks	4	
4 — Mild Dementia	IADL/ability to handle complex task affected	5	
5 — Moderate Dementia	Needs help selecting proper attire		
6 — Moderately Severe Dementia	A) Needs help putting on clothes B) Needs help bathing C) Needs help toileting D) Urinary incontinence E) Fecal incontinence	6 7	
7 – Severe Dementia	A) Speaks 5–6 words a day B) Speaks only 1 word clearly C) Can no longer walk D) Can no longer sit up E) Can no longer smile F) Can no longer hold up head	8	Median survival <6 months for FAST 7 with any of the following 1. Aspiration, upper urinary tract infection, sepsis 2. Multiple stage 3–4 ulcers 3. Persistent fever 4. Weight loss >10% within six months
Note: CFS 9 describes people with life expectancy <6 months who are not otherwise evidently frail			

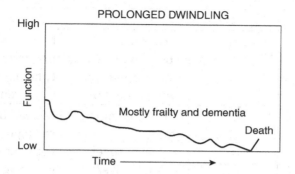

- Towards the end stage, patients suffering from dementia and/or frailty follow a "common pathway" with need for assistance in all basic activities of daily living, functionally dependent in a chair or bed-bound state.
- Functional dependency leads to complications such as pressure ulcers, deep vein thrombosis, infection (urinary tract, chest and skin), constipation, contractures and risk of iatrogenic complications.
- At the end of life, patients have symptoms comparable to those with cancer or other end stage organ diseases including pain, nausea, drowsiness, shortness of breath, fatigue, loss of appetite, demoralization, depression and anxiety.

UNIQUE CHALLENGES FOR PATIENTS WITH DEMENTIA

- Patients with dementia pose unique challenges to providers as they may not be able to describe their symptoms accurately. Often, these patients exhibit behavioral and psychological symptoms of dementia (BPSD) due to unmet care needs such as pain.
- The pain assessment in advanced dementia scale (PAINAD) can be used to evaluate pain severity based on 5 physical observations in patients with dementia.

Observation	0	1	2
Breathing	Normal	Occasional laboured breathing Short period of hyperventilation	Noisy laboured breathing Long period of hyperventilation
Negative vocalization	None	Occasional moan/ groan Low level speech with negative/ disapproving quality	Repeated troubled calling out Loud moaning/ groaning Crying
Facial expression	Smiling or unexpressive	Sad Frightened Frowning	Facial grimacing
Body language	Relaxed	Tense Distressed pacing Fidgeting	Rigid Fists clenched Knees pulled away Pulling or pushing away Striking out
Consolability	No need to console	Distracted or reassured by voice or touch	Unable to console, distract or reassure

- Psychological issues such as depression and anxiety often co-exist with dementia. These may manifest in similar fashion to BPSD and should be assessed with a high index of suspicion. A diagnostic and therapeutic trial with anti-depressants may be necessary.

Management of BPSD	
Personhood management (First line and non-exhaustive)	Management with behavioural medications (Used concurrently with personhood management)
1. Pain assessment and treatment 2. Unmet needs management • Thirst • Hunger • Constipation • Urinary retention • Personal hygiene • Optimized environment for sleep 3. Regular re-orientation 4. Exercise and mobilization 5. Provision of sensory aids (e.g. hearing aids, glasses) 6. Reminiscence therapy 7. Namaste therapy 8. Other meaningful activities based on patient's interest	1. Anti-depressants 2. Psychotropics 3. Sodium valproate
	The neuropsychiatric inventory questionnaire is a useful tool to identify antecedent factors for BPSD such as depression, anxiety, hallucinations, mood lability etc. Note: Behavioural medication usage is associated with complications such as falls and delirium. There is a US FDA "black box" warning for increased mortality from cardiovascular causes in psychotropic usage for BPSD.

DYSPHAGIA AND NUTRITIONAL ISSUES IN DEMENTIA

- Patients with dementia commonly suffer from cognitive dysphagia and develop poor nutritional status. Enteral feeding (via the nasogastric or percutaneous enterostomy routes) has not been proven to reduce the risk of aspiration pneumonia, improve nutritional status, sacral wound healing or prolong survival. Very often, these patients react strongly to insertion of a feeding tube and remove them inadvertently, precipitating the "tube feeding death spiral".
- Careful hand feeding with positioning techniques and good oral hygiene has been shown to be as good as enteral feeding in the relevant

outcomes described above. In most cultures, food and enjoyment of eating play important social and familial functions. Hence, continual efforts to create such meal-time environments will encourage appetite and intake.

- Fluid thickeners and diet modification may be introduced with the intention to decrease risk of aspiration. However, these may be unpalatable to the patient and may increase the risks of dehydration and poor nutritional intake. It is prudent to carefully balance the evidence of risk and benefit, while focusing on treatment individualization.

MANAGEMENT

- Advanced Care Planning.
- Nutritional evaluation and provision of oral nutritional supplementation.
- Physical activity/maintenance program.
  - o Sitting out of bed and therapeutic ambulation to prevent dependency complications.
  - o Active and passive joint movements to maintain mobility and prevent contractures.
- De-prescribe inappropriate medications based on the patient's clinical status, prognosis and values.
- COVID-19 and flu vaccinations.
- Provision of resources for care and social support to maintain patient in the community for as long as possible.
- Caring for the caregivers
  - — Ensure that they are adequately trained and equipped to
    - Maintain hygiene (general and with emphasis on eye, oral, sacrum, skin folds and perineum) for the patient.
    - Feed patients safely.
    - Transfer/bathe patients safely.
  - — They should also receive social and emotional support to prevent burnout.

PRACTICAL TIPS

1. Prognostication in advanced frailty and advanced dementia is still a key research topic. Clinicians can make use of the surprise question to gauge prognosis and plan management.
2. Enteral feeding has not been proven to benefit patients with advanced dementia. Family carers should be engaged in shared decision making, taking into consideration the patient's values and previously stated wishes.
3. Caregivers experience significant stress from caregiving. Engage community resources in the partnership of patient care where appropriate
4. Dignity in end of life care includes:
   - Adequate hygiene.
   - Maintenance of privacy and confidentiality.
   — Giving patients choices as far as possible within safe limits.
   — Being respectful to the person.

REFERENCES

1. Rockwood K, Theou O. Using the clinical frailty scale in allocating scarce health care resources. *Can Geriatr J.* 2020;23(3):210–215.
2. Stow D, Spiers G, Matthews FE, Hanratty B. What is the evidence that people with frailty have needs for palliative care at the end of life? A systematic review and narrative synthesis. *Palliat Med.* 2019;33(4):399–414.
3. American Geriatrics Society Ethics Committee and Clinical Practice and Models of Care Committee. American Geriatrics Society Feeding Tubes in Advanced Dementia Position Statement. *J Am Geriatr Soc.* 2014;62(8): 1590–1593.
4. Dent E, Lien C, Lim WS, *et al.* The Asia-Pacific clinical practice guidelines for the management of frailty [published correction appears in *J Am Med Dir Assoc.* 2018 Jan;19(1):94]. *J Am Med Dir Assoc.* 2017;18(7):564–575.

PAEDIATRIC PALLIATIVE CARE

Chong Poh Heng

INTRODUCTION

If the clinician is asked to attend to a child who may be at risk of dying from a life shortening condition, principles and concepts learnt in previous chapters apply. The difference lies in the attitude and assumptions that one brings to the first consult and subsequent care. These are considered next.

SPECIAL CONSIDERATIONS

- There are inherent differences between adult and children palliative care:
  - Preponderance of non-cancer conditions, with uncertain prognoses and frequent use of technological assistance, like enteral feeding pumps or ventilator support
  - The young person and his/her parents are often 'experts' in their specific illness domain
  - Widespread misconceptions that palliative care is end-of-life care

- In dealing with a 'minor' (<21 years — age of majority), with variable individual neurocognitive development, the approach mandates:
  - understanding nuances around autonomy or self-determination
  - parental rights as proxies or surrogates
  - the clinician's responsibility to guide medical care based on best interest of the child

ASSESSMENT (GENERAL PRINCIPLES)

- History should be obtained from the child wherever feasible. Factors may influence symptom reporting:
  - Pain
  - Culture within which the child situates eg staying stoic
  - Past experiences
  - Not wanting to worry parents
- Use of tools, aids or instruments appropriate to the child's developmental age
- Proxy reporting
  - Listen to, and trust the caregiver, especially parents
- Understand impact on function or life's routines, in relation to play, school, identity, relationships and ambitions of the child
- Implications on the rest in the family
  - Wellbeing and care of siblings
  - How the whole family is kept together as a unit, or otherwise

MANAGEMENT (UNIQUE PERSPECTIVES)

- Interface between active treatments and palliative care
  - 'Best supportive care' (BSC) or transfer of care totally to hospice routine in adult palliative care is uncommon. So is formulation of advance care plans, till late in the course
  - Periodic respite (either at home or at the local inpatient hospice dedicated to caring for these types of children) may help
  - Location of death is mostly the hospital or home, rather than the inpatient hospice

- Treatment strategies
  - Psychological (therapeutic play, visual imagery and art therapy) and physical interventions (splints, acupressure and massage)
  - Two step pain ladder that omits step 2 (avoiding codeine and tramadol in children)
  - Opioid doses may be higher than those in adults, often given intravenously via central lines or using the transmucosal route (instead of subcutaneous injections common in adult practice)
- Psychosocial and spiritual care
  - The parents should own the locus of control as much as possible at this time, as part of shared decision making
  - Need to keep hope 'alive' throughout
  - Bereavement care starts before the child dies and continues for much longer afterwards

PRACTICAL TIPS

1. Impeccable symptom assessment is key to quality care
2. Children who are critically ill have unique needs that need to be acknowledged and incorporated in planning management
3. Parallel planning is a way to manage pervasive uncertainties in children palliative care, and is what most parents would accept (hoping for the best as we plan for the worst)

PAEDIATRIC DRUG FORMULARY (COMMONLY USED DRUGS)

Drug	Indication	Route	Recommended Doses				Times per Day	Notes
			Birth – 1 Month	1 Month – 2 Years	2–12 Years	More Than 12 Years and Adult		
Amitriptyline	Neuropathic pain	Oral		Starting dose 500 microgram – 1 mg/kg/day. Maximum dose 2 mg/kg/day or 150 mg/day in 2 divided doses.		25–50 mg/day; Increase by 10 mg/day every 72 hours until maximum tolerated dose. Maximum dose 150 mg/day in 2 divided doses.	Starting dose given as a single daily dose at night.	Limited experience in very young children. Maximum dose 2 mg/kg/day or 150 mg/day in 2 divided doses.
Bisacodyl	Constipation	Oral			<10 years 5 mg/dose	>10 years 5–10 mg/dose (max. 20 mg)	Single daily dose at night	
		Rectal			<10 years 5 mg/dose Over 10 years 10 mg /dose	10 mg/dose		
Dexamethasone	Symptomatic raised intracranial pressure, intractable vomiting; nerve compression pain	Oral, intravenous or subcutaneous		250 microgram/kg/dose (maximum 16 mg/dose)			Single stat dose followed by maintenance dose as indicated.	Adrenal suppression will occur after 5 days at doses greater than 20 microgram/kg/24 hr Therefore, wean dose to less than 20 microgram/kg/24 hr before stopping.

Drug	Indication	Route			Frequency	Notes
	Intractable vomiting especially associated with chemotherapy	Oral or intravenous		125 microgram/kg/dose (maximum 8 mg/dose)	2 to 3 times in 24 hours	
Diazepam	Status Epilepticus	Per rectum	250–400 microgram/kg/dose OR: Neonates 1.25–2.5 mg/dose; 1 month–2 years 5 mg/dose; 2–12 years 5–10 mg/dose	10 mg/dose	Single dose	Repeat after 10 minutes if necessary
	Spasticity & short-term treatment of anxiety states	Oral	1–12 months 250 microgram/kg/dose (max 2.5 mg/dose); 1–5 years 2.5 mg/dose; 6–12 years 5 mg/dose	10 mg/dose	Start twice daily increasing to 3 or 4 times daily depending on response	Doses of approximately 25–50% of the anti-spasticity doses have been used in breathlessness in palliative care
Diclofenac	Mild to moderate pain; inflammation	Oral, rectal	>6 months 300 microgram – 1 mg/kg/dose	25–50 mg/dose (maximum 150 mg/24hrs)	2–3 times in 24 hours	
Domperidone	Prokinetic antiemetic	Oral	100–300 microgram/kg/dose	200–400 microgram/kg/dose (maximum 20 mg/dose)	3 or 4 times a day. Neonates up to 6.	
		Per rectum	15–35 kg 30 mg/dose/day & >35 kg 60 mg/dose/day	60 mg/day	2–3 divided doses in 24 hours	

(Continued)

(Continued)

Drug	Indication	Route	Recommended Doses				Times per day	Notes
			Birth – 1 month	1 month – 2 years	2–12 years	More Than 12 years and adult		
Gabapentin	Neuropathic pain	Oral		10 mg/kg once daily for 1–4 days, then twice daily for 1–4 days, then three times daily maximum 20 mg/kg/dose		300 mg once daily for 1–4 days; then 300 mg twice daily for 1–4 days; then 300 mg three times daily. Increase as tolerated to maximum 600 mg three times daily	Up to 3 times in 24 hours	Adverse effects can be reduced by slower dose titration
Haloperidol	Nausea and vomiting particularly biochemical causes; antipsychotic (minimal sedation)	Oral		25–50 microgram/kg/dose (max 5 mg)		1.5–5 mg/dose	Once at night or twice daily	
		Intravenous or subcutaneous continuous infusion		25–50 microgram/kg/24 hrs (max 5 mg)		1.5–5 mg/24 hrs	Continuous infusion over 24 hours	

Drug	Indication	Route		Paediatric dose	Adult dose	Frequency	Notes
Hyoscine butylbromide	Symptomatic relief of pain due to smooth muscle spasm	Oral		150–300 microgram/kg/dose Maximum doses: up to 5 years: 5 mg/dose 6–12 years: 10 mg/dose	10–20 mg/dose	3–4 times in 24 hours	
	Excess respiratory tract secretions, colic due to inoperable bowel obstructtion	Intravenous or subcutaneous continuous infection		300–1800 microgram/kg/24 hrs Maximum doses: up to 5 years: 30 mg/24 hrs 6–12 years: 60 mg/24 hrs	40–120 mg/24 hrs for bowel obstruction	Continuous infusion over 24 hours	
Ibuprofen	Nonsteroidal anti-inflammatory drug for mild/moderate pain	Oral		5–10 mg/kg/dose (Maximum 30 mg/kg/24 hrs or 2.4 g/24 hrs)	200–400 mg/dose (Maximum 2.4 g/24 hrs)	3–4 times in 24 hours	
Lactulose	Osmotic laxative	Oral		1 month–1 year 2.5 ml/dose 1–5 years 5 ml/dose 5–10 years 10 ml/dose	15 ml/dose	Two doses in 24 hours	May cause excess flatus and colic at higher doses
Lorazepam	Acute dyspnoea and anxiety attacks	Intravenous, subcutaneous, or sublingual		20–50 microgram/kg/dose	1–4 mg/dose	PRN max 4 times	

(Continued)

(Continued)

Drug	Indication	Route	Recommended Doses Birth – 1 month	1 month – 2 years	2–12 years	More Than 12 years and adult	Times per day	Notes
Metoclopramide	Nausea and vomiting especially due to delayed gastric emptying	Oral		100 microgram/kg/dose maximum single doses: <3 years 1 mg; 3–5 years 2 mg; 6–9 years 2.5 mg; >9 years 5 mg		10 mg/dose	PRN up to 8 hourly	
		Intravenous or subcutaneous continuous infusion		300–500 microgram/kg/24 hrs (maximum 30 mg/24 hrs)		300–500 microgram/kg/24 hrs Doses up to 100 mg/24 hrs in delayed gastric emptying	Continuous infusion over 24 hours	
Midazolam	Agitation or anxiety in end-of-life care. Status epilepticcus	Buccal or sublingual		200–300 microgram/kg/dose		10 mg/dose	PRN max 6–8 hourly	If more than 2 doses are required in 24 hours, consider continuous infusion
	Agitation or anxiety in end-of-life care	Intravenous or subcutaneous injection		50–100 microgram/kg/dose (maximum 5 mg)		5 mg/dose	PRN – repeat up to hourly	If more than 2 doses are required in 24 hours, consider continuous infusion

	Agitation or anxiety in end-of-life care	Intravenous or subcutaneous infusion	240–420 microgram/kg/24 hrs	25–60 mg/24 hrs	Continuous infusion over 24 hours	If patient does not settle on 30 mg/24 hours or 420 microgram/kg/24 hrs, add in anti-psychotic before increasing dose further
Morphine	Strong opioid	Oral or rectal	1–3 months 50–100 microgram/kg/dose 3–6 months 100–150 microgram/kg/dose 6–12 months 200 microgram/kg/dose 1–12 years 200–300 microgram/kg/dose (max. 15 mg) >12 years 10–15 mg/dose		PRN — usual frequency is 4–6 hourly; maximum hourly.	Always prescribe regular stimulant laxatives. For dyspnoea or intractable cough, doses of approximately 50% of analgesic doses are effective.
		Intravenous or subcutaneous continuous injection	Birth–3 months 50–75 microgram/kg/dose 3–6 months 75 microgram/kg/dose 6–12 months 100 microgram/kg/dose Over 12 months 100–150 microgram/kg/dose (maximum 7.5 mg/dose)	5–7.5 mg/dose	PRN. Usual frequency is 4–6 hourly; maximum hourly in titration of analgesia.	

(Continued)

(Continued)

Drug	Indication	Route	Birth – 1 month	1 month – 2 years	2–12 years	More Than 12 years and adult	Times per day	Notes
Macrogols (Movicol paediatric plain or Movicol half)	Osmotic laxative; Chronic constipation	Oral			1–6 years 1–8 sachets/24 hours 6–12 years 2–12 sachets/24 hours	2–16 sachets/24 hours	Total dose over 24-hour period.	Constipation, including opioid-induced. Start at low dose and increase according to response. Faecal impaction. Start at low dose and increase by 2 sachets per 24 hours until bowels open. Then halve dose and continue as maintenance.
Ondansetron	Nausea and vomiting associated with chemotherapy or radiotherapy;	Subcutaneous or intravenous injection			150 microgram/kg/dose (maximum 4 mg/dose)	8 mg/dose	PRN max 3 times daily or total daily dose as continuous infusion over 24 hours.	Oral bioavailability is approximately 50%. Pruritis doses are equivalent.
	opiate induced pruritis.	Oral			1–12 years 4 mg/dose	8 mg/dose	2–3 times in 24 hours	

	Indication	Route				
Omeprazole	Gastrooesophageal reflux; treatment and prophylaxis of peptic ulcer disease including that associated with NSAID administration	Oral or intravenous		1 month–2 years 0.7–3 mg/kg/dose (max 20 mg) once daily OR 10–20 kg 10 mg/dose once daily increased if necessary, to 20 mg/dose once daily >20 kg 20 mg/dose once daily increased if necessary, to 40 mg/dose once daily	40 mg/dose	Once daily
Paracetamol	Mild to moderate pain; pyrexia	Oral, rectal or intravenous	<3 months 10–15 mg/kg/dose (maximum 60 mg/kg/24 hours)	10–20 mg/kg/dose <6 months Max. 60 mg/kg/24 hrs >6 months Max. 90 mg/kg/24 hrs	500 mg–1 g/dose maximum 4 g/24 hrs	4–6 times in 24 hours
Senna (7.5 mg tablets)	Stimulant laxative	Oral		0.5 ml/kg/dose (max 2.5 ml)	2–6 years: 1/2 to 1 tablet/dose 6–12 years: 1–2 tablets/dose	2–4 tablets/dose	Single dose at night

REFERENCES

1. Additional resources (free) for learners can be found at the International Children's Palliative Care Network website. http://www.icpcn.org/icpcns-elearning-programme/
2. Downing J (editor). *Children's Palliative Care: An International Case-Based Manual*. Springer; 2020.
3. A comprehensive drug formulary is available (free) at the Together for Short Lives (UK) website https://www.togetherforshortlives.org.uk/resource/appm-master-formulary-2020-5th-edition/

SECTION 4: TERMINAL SYMPTOMS

NUTRITION AND HYDRATION

Chau Mo Yee

INTRODUCTION

The role of artificial hydration and nutrition at the end of life is controversial for patients, families, and palliative care providers. While the provision of food and water is fundamental for human survival, its provision by artificial means near the end of life may not prolong life. In fact, it may worsen suffering by causing increased secretions and dyspnoea.

DEFINITION

Artificial nutrition and hydration may be defined as nutritional and hydration support of an invasive nature requiring the placement of a tube into the alimentary tract or parenterally via intravenous or subcutaneous means.

Concerns About Withholding Nutrition and Hydration at the End of Life

- *"The patient will die hungry"*:
  - Explain to families that anorexia and decreased oral intake is part of the normal process of dying from a terminal illness. Consequently, patients near the end of life rarely express hunger.

- *"The patient's mouth and lips are dry"*:
  — Sensations of dry mouth can be relieved by regular oral care, lubricants (like Bioxtra or Biotene) and ice chips. This symptom is not relieved by parenteral hydration. Pleasure feeding is allowed if the patient is alert enough to take orally.

Disadvantages of Artificial Nutrition and Hydration

For many patients near the end of life, the burdens of artificial hydration and nutrition (AHN) may outweigh the benefits.

- Potential harm:
  — Fluid overload, due to low plasma protein level, leads to peripheral edema, ascites, pulmonary edema, increased throat secretions (terminal rattling) and vomiting.
  — Complications and problems associated with the use of invasive tubes or cannulas may arise.
- Limited benefits:
  — In studies of patients at the terminal phase of life, there is no evidence that AHN improves quality of life, diminishes suffering or extends survival.

PRACTICAL TIPS

1. Decisions about the use of hydration and nutrition must be made on an individual basis, carefully weighing the risks and benefits of intervention and non-intervention.
2. Communication
   - The topic of AHN should be raised by the clinician routinely with patients and families at the terminal phase of life.
   - Clinicians should seek to understand the perspectives of patients and families and communicate the potential risk and uncertainties involved.
   - The families' distress and desire to express love to the patients should be validated. Clinicians can redirect them to what can be done to show care for the patients eg oral care, skin care, physical touch etc.

3. If unable to reach a consensus, a time-limited trial of therapy may be considered, with frequent reassessment and the understanding to discontinue therapy if symptoms worsen eg. SC Normal Saline 0.5–1 L/day.
4. Discuss advance care plans before patient becomes terminally ill.

REFERENCES

1. Kingdon A, Spathis A, Brodrick R, *et al*. What is the impact of clinically assisted hydration in the last days of life? A systematic literature review and narrative synthesis. *BMJ Support Palliat Care*. 2021;11(1):68–74 doi:10.1136/bmjspcare-2020-002600
2. Bruera E, Hui D, Dalal S, Torres-Vigil I, Trumble J, Roosth J, *et al*. Parenteral hydration in patients with advanced cancer: a multicenter, double-blind, placebo-controlled randomized trial. *J Clin Oncol*. 2013;31(1):111–118. doi: 10.1200/JCO.2012.44.6518
3. Fritzson A, Tavelin B, Axelsson B. Association between parenteral fluids and symptoms in hospital end-of-life care: An observational study of 280 patients. *BMJ Support Palliat Care*. 2015;5:160–168. doi:10.1136/bmjspcare-2013-000501

PALLIATIVE SEDATION

Poi Choo Hwee

INTRODUCTION

Palliative sedation is the controlled administration of sedative medications to reduce patient consciousness to the extent necessary to render *refractory* suffering tolerable. The aim of palliative sedation is the relief of symptoms and not the shortening of life in a patient who has a progressive and irreversible life-threatening illness, and is actively or imminently *dying*.

Refractory suffering occurs when symptoms "cannot be adequately controlled despite aggressive efforts to identify tolerable therapy that does not compromise consciousness". A symptom is regarded as refractory when all possible treatments cannot provide adequate symptom relief, when treatment is associated with excessive and unacceptable side-effects, or when treatment is unlikely to achieve relief within a tolerable time frame. Refractory symptoms may include pain, delirium, agitation, restlessness and dyspnea.

'Imminently' *dying* refers to patients who will probably die within hours to days. It usually means a prognosis of death within 14 days.

There are concerns that palliative sedation may hasten death, but there are no conclusive studies to show that it worsens survival.

INDICATIONS FOR PALLIATIVE SEDATION

Sedation may be indicated for patients with refractory or intractable suffering due to physical symptoms, when there are a lack of other methods for palliation within an acceptable time frame without unacceptable adverse effects.

The most common symptoms include:

- Agitated delirium
- Intractable and severe dyspnea
- Overwhelming pain crisis
- Uncontrolled seizures
- Intractable nausea and vomiting
- Emergency situations, including massive haemorrhage, asphyxia or stridor

Palliative sedation for severe non-physical symptoms, including refractory depression, anxiety, demoralisation and existential distress remains contentious.

TYPES OF SEDATION

The aim of palliative sedation is to provide relief from intolerable and intractable symptoms. As the goal is symptom relief and not unconsciousness, clinicians should use the lowest possible effective dose of sedatives to achieve symptom control (proportionality).

The level of sedation should be balanced in accordance to patient/surrogate's perceived level of symptom relief, burden of adverse effects and the ability to interact meaningfully. Intermittent or mild sedation should generally be attempted first. For some patients, the sedation dose is small enough to maintain the patient's ability to communicate and still provide adequate relief without a total loss of interactive function.

Continuous deep sedation could be selected if:

1. Suffering is intense and intolerable
2. Suffering is refractory
3. Death is anticipated within hours or a few days

4. Patient's wish is explicit
5. Catastrophic event at the end of life such as massive haemorrhage or asphyxia

EVALUATION BEFORE INITIATING PALLIATIVE SEDATION

A complete patient evaluation should be done, which includes:

- Patient's medical history, physical examination and all relevant investigations
- Psychosocial, spiritual evaluation
- Prognosis
- Patient's capacity to make decisions about on-going care

PROCESSES BEFORE INITIATING PALLIATIVE SEDATION

- Active involvement of patient and family/surrogate in the decision-making process: discuss limited prognosis, therapeutic options (benefits and risks), goals of care discussion (including DNR order) and care goals
- Discuss the risks and benefits of artificial nutrition and hydration
- Presence of a DNR order
- Involvement of 2 independent palliative care physicians in the assessment
- Interdisciplinary evaluation: eg. Primary specialists, nurses or social workers
- Consider consulting the hospital ethics and legal departments if indicated (ie presence of conflict with patient, patient's family or healthcare professional regarding the use of palliative sedation)

MEDICATIONS USED FOR PALLIATIVE SEDATION

- Midazolam 1–2.5 mg SC/IV stat and continuous infusion 0.5–2 mg/hr
  — Doses can be titrated up to 5–10 mg/hr proportionately to achieve sedation
  — May cause paradoxical agitation

- Phenobarbitone 200 mg IV/SC bolus and continuous infusion at 600 mg/day (Maintenance dose: 600–1600 mg/ day)

PATIENT MONITORING & CARE

- Review regularly until symptom control is achieved with the initiation of palliative sedation
- Daily review of the dose of sedatives, with the aim to use the minimum dose necessary for symptom relief
- Daily review of the risks and benefits of artificial nutrition and hydration
- May discontinue heart rate, blood pressure and temperature monitoring if goal of care is to ensure comfort
- Maintain good nursing care: oral care, eye care, skin care and pressure wound care
- Continue providing regular updates and emotional support to the family

PRACTICAL TIPS

1. The decision to initiate palliative sedation should only be undertaken when physical symptoms are intractable and when treatment measures have failed to adequately control symptoms.
2. It should only be carried out after a thorough clinical assessment and discussion between the patient, family, primary specialists and other members of the multi-disciplinary team.
3. A Palliative care specialist should be consulted before initiating palliative sedation.

REFERENCES

1. Claessens P, Menten. Palliative sedation: A review of the research literature. *J Pain Symptom Manage.* 2008;36:310–333.
2. Kirk TW, Mahon MM; Palliative Sedation Task Force. National Hospice and Palliative Care Organization (NHPCO) Position Statement and Commentary on the Use of Palliative Sedation in Imminently Dying Terminally Ill Patients. *J Pain Symptom Manage.* 2010;39(5):914–923.

3. Cherny NI, Radbruch L. Board of the European Association for Palliative Care. European Association for Palliative Care (EAPC) recommended framework for the use of sedation in palliative care. *Palliat Med.* 2009;23: 581–593.

4. De Graeff A, Dean M. Palliative sedation therapy in the last weeks of life: A literature review and recommendations for standards. *J Palliat Med.* 2007; 10(1):67–85. doi:10.1089/jpm.2006.0139

5. Maltoni M, Scarpi E, Rosati M, *et al.* Palliative sedation in end-of-life care and survival: A systematic review [published correction appears in *J Clin Oncol.* 2012 Sep 20;30(27):3429]. *J Clin Oncol.* 2012;30(12):1378–1383. doi:10.1200/JCO.2011.37.3795

6. Bodnar J. A Review of agents for palliative sedation/continuous deep sedation: Pharmacology and practical applications, *J Pain Palliat Care Pharmacother.* 2017;31:1,16–37, DOI: 10.1080/15360288.2017.1279502

TERMINAL SECRETIONS

Chau Mo Yee

INTRODUCTION

Terminal or respiratory tract secretions are common in the terminal phase of life, occurring in up to 23–95% of patients at the end of life. While there is no evidence that patients find this symptom disturbing, it may be distressing to the family and caregivers. The presence of terminal secretions is a good predictor of impending death, with a prognosis of short days.

CAUSES

As dying patients become increasingly unconscious, they lose their ability to swallow and clear oral secretions. As air moves over the pooled secretions in the oropharynx and bronchi, the resulting turbulence may cause rattling noises. The airway obstruction leads to the production of more secretions, aggravating the terminal secretions.

Two sub-types of terminal secretions have been proposed, although the significance relating to treatment has not yet been established.

Type 1	• Salivary secretions accumulate when the swallowing reflexes are inhibited and the cough reflex is ineffective
Type 2	• Bronchial secretions caused by a pulmonary pathology and/or other pathologies which cannot be coughed up or swallowed

MANAGEMENT

Non-Pharmacological

- Position the patient on their side or in a semi-prone position to facilitate postural drainage
- Ensure good mouth care
- Reduce use of parenteral fluids to prevent overhydration

Note: Most secretions are usually below the larynx and inaccessible to suctioning. It is also very uncomfortable for patients. Routine use of deep suctioning should be discouraged.

Pharmacological

Anti-muscarinic/anti-cholinergic drugs are used to reduce formation of new secretions.

- Hyoscine Butylbromide (Buscopan) 20 mg SC PRN
  — Continuous infusion at 40–120 mg/day
  — Buscopan does not cross the blood-brain barrier
- Hyoscine Hydrobromide (Scopolamine) 400 mcg SC PRN
  — Continuous infusion 800–2400 mcg/day
  — Scopolamine crosses the blood-brain barrier and causes sedation
- Glycopyrrolate 400 mcg SC PRN
  — Continuous infusion 800–2400 mcg/day
  — Rarely causes delirium or sedation as it does not cross the blood brain barrier
- Atropine 1% eyedrops 1–2 drops q 4–6 hourly can also be given sublingually
  — Mydriasis, tachycardia, arrhythmia, constipation, urinary retention and dry mouth

Frequent assessment for efficacy and adverse effects of pharmacological treatment is needed

PRACTICAL TIPS

1. Anti-cholinergic drugs should be used at the first sign of terminal secretions.

2. Communication
   - If reducing or discontinuing fluid intake is used as one of the strategies to reduce secretions, it is important to communicate this to the family, while addressing their concerns about hydration and nutrition at the end of life.
   - Discuss with the patient's families about the cause, implications and their fears and concerns about terminal secretions to allay their distress.
   - It is important to prepare families about the short prognosis that may be associated with terminal secretions.

REFERENCES

1. Wildiers H, Menten J. Death rattle: Prevalence, prevention and treatment. *J Pain Symptom Manage.* 2002;23:310–317.
2. Wee B, Hillier R. Interventions for noisy breathing in patients near to death. *Cochrane Database Syst Rev* 2008;1:CD005177.
3. Lokker ME, van Zuylen L, van der Rijt CC, van der Heide A. Prevalence, impact, and treatment of death rattle: A systematic review. *J Pain Symptom Manage* 2014;47:105–122.Tatusapi endandu cipsum quis ut ommodit aerate est reprepe rfernate escius eos sum ex estis mintiatemosa quosam, nullupt aquam, con re natem resti con rerferum am dolorios vendignimusa non el min pe et quo ma et et ut adi volupta eptiassiti utem id et alia cus dessit,
4. van Esch HJ, van Zuylen L, Geijteman ECT, et al. Effect of prophylactic subcutaneous scopolamine butylbromide on death rattle in patients at the end of life: The SILENCE Randomized Clinical Trial. *JAMA.* 2021;326(13):1268–1276.

SECTION 5: PALLIATIVE CARE EMERGENCIES

ACUTE PAIN CRISIS

Allyn Hum and Raphael Lee

Allyn Hum and Raphael Lee

INTRODUCTION

An acute pain crisis is a palliative care emergency. It is defined as intolerable, uncontrolled pain which causes severe distress to the patient, family or both. The physical pain is often scored at $\geq 7/10$ on the NRS (Numeric Rating Scale) and the patient is obviously very distressed by it. Its frequency varies depending on definitions and was described at 15% in one study.

CAUSES

It can occur suddenly, as in the case of an acute pathological fracture or as an exacerbation of background chronic pain.

MANAGEMENT

Principles of Management

- Respond by being present as soon as able
- Make a rapid clinical assessment as to the aetiology of the pain, and its nature
- Establish the intensity of the pain experienced, using verbal descriptors or the numerical rating scale
- Determine analgesics used thus far, and the patient's response to the medications

- Use strong opioids in a pain crisis
  - Select the opioid based on an understanding of the nature of the pain. The mode of administration should be parenteral to achieve rapid pain relief
- Maintain a continuous infusion of the opioid, or increase the baseline opioid infusion to maintain analgesia

PHARMACOLOGICAL

A Patient Who Is Opioid-Naïve

- Morphine 2.5 mg IV (every 5–10 min) or 2.5 mg SC (every 15–30 min) OR
- Fentanyl 20 mcg IV (every 5–10 min) or 20 mcg SC (every 15–30 min) or till analgesia* is achieved

A Patient Already on Oral Opioids

- Convert to equivalent parenteral dose, e.g. a patient on Morphine 90 mg/day PO (= parenteral 30 mg/day)
- Administer Morphine at 1/10th of the daily dose, 3 mg IV (every 5–10 min) or 3 mg SC (every 15–30 min) till analgesia* is achieved
- If ineffective after 3 doses, increase to 1/6th of the daily dose, 5 mg IV (every 5–10 min) or 5 mg SC (every 15–30 min) till analgesia* is achieved

ON PARENTERAL OPIOIDS

- Administer at 1/10th of the total daily dose
  e.g. a patient on Fentanyl 25 mcg/hr (= 600 mcg/day) – Fentanyl 60 mcg IV (every 5–10 min) or Fentanyl 60 mcg SC (every 15–30 min) till analgesia* is achieved)
- If ineffective after 3 doses, increase to 1/6th of the daily dose (Fentanyl 100 mcg IV (every 5–10 min) or Fentanyl 100 mcg SC (every 15–30 min) till analgesia* is achieved)

  *Pain is reduced by >50% by verbal assessment or NRS.

ADJUVANTS

NMDA Antagonists

- Ketamine can be considered in patients with severe cancer neuropathic pain particularly if associated with features of the "wind up phenomenon" and central sensitisation
- Refractoriness to opioids or in combination with an adjuvant

Na Channel Blockers

- Parenteral Lignocaine has shown modest effect in opioid refractory pain with a neuropathic component

PRACTICAL TIPS

1. Once the pain crisis is addressed, consider adjusting the baseline opioid dose. If pain is predominantly neuropathic, consider the use of, or optimisation of adjuvant agents.
2. If appropriate, consider interventional techniques (e.g. nerve blocks) to aid in the relief of pain.
3. Anxiety can increase the experience of suffering and should be addressed with the use of benzodiazepines given via the parenteral route during such episodes.
4. Obtain the help of the palliative and/or pain team.

REFERENCES

1. Moryl N, Foley KM. Managing an acute pain crisis in a patient with advanced cancer. "This is as much of a crisis as a code". *JAMA*. 2008;299(12):1457–1467.
2. Mercadante S, Villari P, Ferrera P, Casuccio A, Fulfaro F. Rapid titration with intravenous morphine for severe cancer pain and immediate oral conversion. *Cancer*. 2002 Jul 1;95(1):203–208.
3. Chia SC, Hum A, Ong W, Lee A, Parenteral lignocaine in cancer neuropathic pain: A series of case reports. *Prog Pallia Care*. 2014;22:253–257.
4. Bell RF, Eccleston C, Kalso EA. Ketamine as an adjuvant to opioids for cancer pain. *Cochrane Database Syst Rev*. 2017;6(6):CD003351.

AIRWAY OBSTRUCTION (STRIDOR)

Yee Choon Meng

INTRODUCTION

Stridor is an abnormal, high-pitched breath sound caused by blockage in the throat or larynx. It is usually heard during inspiration. It can be very distressing to both patients and their families.

CAUSES

- Carcinomas of the upper airway (e.g. laryngeal or nasopharyngeal carcinoma)
- Intra-luminal obstruction of the trachea due to lung or oesophageal cancers
- External compression by tumour, metastasis or mediastinal lymphadenopathy
- Recurrent laryngeal nerve palsy (from stroke/metastasis from lung cancer)

TREATMENT

Non-Pharmacological

- Consider emergency interventional bronchoscopy for intra-luminal stenting, laser/cryotherapy or brachytherapy if feasible
- Consider emergency tracheostomy if this is in keeping with the trajectory of illness and goals of care

- Reduce fluids and nasogastric (NG) feeding significantly (<500 ml/day) in view of risk of secretions

Pharmacological

- Dexamethasone 16–24 mg PO/IV may help to reduce laryngeal oedema
- Morphine IV/SC if the patient is dyspnoeic (See the chapter on Dyspnea)
- Buscopan 20 mg PRN SC up to Q4H for throat secretions

PRACTICAL TIPS

1. If stridor is not reversible and the patient is not for tracheostomy, discuss palliative sedation with the family (consult the palliative care team).
2. For patients with stroke and bilateral vocal cord palsy, the stridor may resolve with a trial of dexamethasone.
3. Continuous Positive Airway Pressure has been reported to be useful for selected cases.
4. Nebulised Adrenaline 1:1000 (dilute into 5 ml N/S) has been used in cases of steroid-resistant stridor.

REFERENCES

1. Flockton R, Ellenshaw J. Use of nebulised adrenaline in the management of steroid-resistant stridor. *Palliat Med.* 2007;21:723–724.
2. Ma CM. Major airway obstruction. *Newslett HK Soc Palliat Med.* 2010 Apr:10–11.
3. Okiror L. Bronchoscopic management of patients with symptomatic airway stenosis and prognostic factors for survival. *Ann Thorac Surg.* 2015;99: 1725–1730

4. Lee J. The use of continuous positive airway pressure ventilation in the palliative management of stridor in a head and neck cancer patient. *J Pain Symptom Manage.* 2019;58:e3–e5.

BLEEDING

Yee Choon Meng and Joseph Ong

Yee Choon Meng and Joseph Ong

INTRODUCTION

Some cancers form very vascular tumours that can bleed easily. Bleeding may also occur in patients with leukaemia, myelodysplasia, thrombocytopenia or if they are on anticoagulant therapy. Bleeding occurs in 6–10% of cancers. The management of bleeding depends on the site that is involved.

A 'terminal bleeding' event can be traumatic for patients, families and healthcare providers involved.

MANAGEMENT

1. Anticipate and prepare
   • Identify and optimise risk factors
   • Consider patient's prognosis, functional status, and goals of care
2. Manage the event, especially if massive bleed
   • Assure the patient
   • Be there — stay with the patient, and
   • Comfort, calm, camouflage bleeding with dark towels
   • Consider anxiolytics if terminal
3. After the event
   • Provide practical and psychological support to those involved including relatives and staff

General Measures

- Apply pressure if anatomically possible with appropriate material (e.g. gauze/gamgee pads)
- Sedate if terminal event (e.g. stat SC/IM midazolam 5 mg)

Specific Measures

Local
- Pack with appropriate material (e.g. gauze with adrenaline/tranexamic acid/sucralfate or calcium alginate dressing for skin/mouth/rectum/vagina)
  — Adrenaline 1:1000
  — Tranexamic acid (500 mg in 5 ml water)
  — Sucralfate suspension (2 g in 10 ml) or paste
Systemic
- Identify and discontinue offending agents e.g. anticoagulant, antiplatelet agents.
- Vitamin K 10 mg IV daily for 3 days if appropriate
- Tranexamic acid 500 mg – 1 g TDS PO/IV
  Relative contraindications:
  — Patients with risk factors for stroke/emboli/cardiovascular event/hypercoagulable states
  — Dose-adjustment required in patients with renal impairment

Nasal/Oropharynx

Nasal
- Anterior: silver nitrate stick, local tranexamic acid
- Posterior: vasoconstrictors (e.g. phenylephrine, oxymetazoline, topical cocaine), nasal sponge tampon (Merocel)
Oral cavity
- Haemostatic sponge (e.g. Surgicel/Gelfoam)
- Mouth wash: tranexamic acid (5 g in 50 ml warm water BD) or sucralfate suspension (2 g/10 ml suspension BD)
- Nebulized adrenaline (2.5–5 ml 1% in 5 ml saline QDS)

Respiratory Tract

- Rule out pulmonary embolism
- Suppress cough
- Possibly nebulized tranexamic acid 500 mg/5 ml QDS

Upper Gastro-Intestinal Tract

- Proton pump inhibitors
- Octreotide (SC/IV 100–200 mcg TDS or 600 mcg over 24 hr) or Somatostatin 250 mcg/hr IV

Urinary Tract

Urinary bladder
- Consider continuous bladder washout
  — For haemorrhagic cystitis, intermittent bladder irrigation with saline may help
- Intravesical administration of antifibrinolytics
  — Alum 1% (50 g in 5 L saline), irrigate bladder at 250 ml/hr
  — Silver nitrate solution 0.5–1.0% instilled over 10–20 min has also been used intra-vesically to cause chemical cauterisation and eschar formation. However, it may induce painful bladder spasms
  — Avoid tranexamic acid as there is a risk of clot retention

In prostate cancer, insertion of a Foley catheter with mild traction may halt bleeding.

PRACTICAL TIPS

1. Consider radiotherapy, arterial embolization or endoscopy (including bronchoscopy, cystoscopy) for direct haemostasis if appropriate.
2. Prepare family members for the possibility of a terminal bleeding event in a sensitive manner so as not to invoke fear. Educate caregivers on how to deliver fast-acting sedatives from an emergency kit if needed, as well as the importance of dark sheets, towels, and

clothing to reduce the visibility of blood. As these events can be traumatic for staff and family members, there may be a need to debrief after the event.

REFERENCES

1.   Harris DG, Noble SI. Management of terminal haemorrhage in patients with advanced cancer: A systematic literature review. *J Pain Symptom Manage.* 2009;38(6):913–927.
2.   Sood R, Mancinetti M, Betticher D, Cantin B, Ebneter A. Management of bleeding in palliative care patients in the general internal medicine ward: A systematic review. *Ann Med Surg (Lond).* 2020;50:14–23.

HYPERCALCEMIA

Lee Chung Seng

INTRODUCTION

Hypercalcemia occurs in 20–30% of patients with cancer. Patients with hypercalcemia of malignancy often have a poor prognosis with 50% of patients dying within 30 days.

Hypercalcemia occurs when corrected serum (ionised) calcium levels are >2.6 mmol/L.

Mild Hypercalcemia	2.6–2.9 mmol/L
Moderate Hypercalcemia	3.0–3.4 mmol/L
Severe Hypercalcemia	>3.5 mmol/L

There are 3 major mechanisms that cause hypercalcemia in cancer patients:

1. Tumour secretion of parathyroid hormone-related protein (PTHrP)
2. Osteolytic metastases with a local release of cytokines (osteoclast activating factors)
3. Tumour production of 1,25-dihydroxyvitamin D (Calcitriol)

CLINICAL FEATURES

General	• Dehydration, polydipsia, polyuria, pruritus
Gastrointestinal	• Anorexia, nausea, vomiting, constipation, ileus
Neurological	• Fatigue, lethargy, muscle weakness, hypo-reflexia, confusion, psychosis, seizure, drowsiness, coma
Cardiac	• Bradycardia, prolonged P-R, shortened Q-T, wide T-waves, arrhythmias

CAUSES (CANCERS)

- Breast
- Lung
- Multiple Myeloma and Lymphoma
- Head and Neck
- Renal

The most common cancers associated with hypercalcemia are breast and lung cancers as well as multiple myeloma and lymphoma.

MANAGEMENT

Pharmacological

General Management

- Discontinue drugs which may precipitate hypercalcemia (Calcium/ Vit D, Calcitriol, Thiazides, Antacids)
- Treat underlying disease if possible
- Aggressive IV hydration (2–3 L/day), with a judiciously reduced volume in the elderly or those at risk of fluid overload

Specific Management

- Bisphosphonates
  — Ensure that the patient is adequately hydrated before starting Bisphosphonates

- — Use Pamidronate IV (30–90 mg in 500 ml normal saline over 2–4 hr) or Zoledronic acid (4 mg over 15–30 min)
- — Repeat calcium levels after Bisphosphonate administration only after 4–7 days
- — Repeated doses of Bisphosphonates can be given only one week after for recalcitrant hypercalcemia
- — Side-effects may include flu-like symptoms (fever, arthralgias, myalgia, fatigue, bone pain), hypocalcemia, hypophosphatemia, impaired renal function and osteonecrosis of the jaw (rare)
- — For dosing in renal impairment, ensure adequate hydration with saline and treat with a reduced dosage/slower infusion rate (i.e. 30 mg of Pamidronate over 4 hr)
- Calcitonin
  - — SC 4–8 IU/kg; every 6–12 hr x 2 days
  - — Efficacy is limited to the first 48 hr due to the development of tachyphylaxis (receptor downregulation)
  - — Reduction in calcium levels is usually minimal and temporary
- Denosumab
  - — Human monoclonal antibody to RANKL, working through decreasing osteoclast activity and bone resorption
  - — An alternative option for patients with hypercalcemia that is refractory to zoledronic acid or in severe renal impairment when bisphosphonates are contraindicated
  - — SC 60–120mg and dose should not be repeated earlier than one week following the administration
  - — In renal impairment, may consider lower dose to avoid hypocalcemia
  - — Side effects may include bone pain, nausea, diarrhoea, shortness of breath and in rare instances, osteonecrosis of the jaw
- Steroids are only recommended for corticosteroid sensitive cancers like myeloma and lymphoma that produce 1,25-dihydroxyvitamin D
- Dialysis is generally not used for advanced cancer patients with malignant hypercalcemia

PRACTICAL TIPS

1. Zoledronate is more potent than Pamidronate and can be given over a much shorter time.

2. The use of Frusemide for the correction of hypercalcemia is no longer recommended.
3. Denosumab is an option for patients with hypercalcemia that is refractory to zoledronic acid or in severe renal impairment when bisphosphonates are contraindicated.

REFERENCES

1. Penel N, Dewas S. Cancer-associated hypercalcemia treated by intravenous bisphosphonates: A survival and prognostic factor analysis. *Support Care Cancer*. 2008;16:387–392.
2. Major P, Lortholary A. Zoledronic acid is superior to pamidronate in the treatment of hypercalcaemia of malignancy: A pooled analysis of two randomized, controlled clinical trials. *J Clin Oncol*. 2001;19(2):558–567.
3. Stewart AF. Hypercalcaemia associated with malignancy. *New Engl J Med*. 2005;352:(4):373–379.
4. Hu MI, Glezerman IG, Leboulleux S, Insogna K, Gucalp R, Misiorowski W, *et al*. Denosumab for treatment of hypercalcemia of malignancy. *J Clin Endocrinol Metab*. 2014;99:3144–3152.
5. Adhikaree J, Newby Y, Sundar S. Denosumab should be the treatment of choice for bisphosphonate refractory hypercalcaemia of malignancy. *BMJ Case Rep*. 2014; 2014:bcr2013202861.
6. Hu MI, Glezerman I, Leboulleux S, Insogna K, Gucalp R, Misiorowski W, *et al*. Denosumab for patients with persistent or relapsed hypercalcemia of malignancy despite recent bisphosphonate treatment. *J Natl Cancer Inst*. 2013;105:1417–1420.

SEIZURES

Yee Choon Meng and Joseph Ong

Seizures are common in patients with end-stage disease, occurring in a variety of conditions and are significant sources of distress for patients and families.

Although the actual incidence of seizures in palliative settings is not known, it is estimated that they occur between 49–85% in those with primary brain tumours, and around 24% in those with brain metastases [most common with melanoma (67%) and least with breast cancer (16%)]. Paraneoplastic encephalitis is another potential cause of seizures in patients with systemic cancer. Other aetiologies common at the end of life include metabolic encephalopathies such as hyponatraemia or hypoglycaemia, infections, or side effects of therapy.

The common types of seizures seen in palliative care patients are generalised tonic-clonic and simple partial seizures affecting one side of the body. Consider also the possibility of non-convulsive status epilepticus which can occur in the absence of intracranial lesions.

In order to avoid significant morbidity and refractory status, an accepted operational definition of status epilepticus would be:

- Continuous seizures of ≥5 minutes in tonic–clonic seizures and ≥10 min in focal impaired awareness seizures, or

147

- ≥2 discrete seizures between which there is incomplete recovery of consciousness

CAUSES

- Brain metastasis or primary brain tumour
- Hypoglycaemia, hyponatraemia, uraemia
- Hepatic encephalopathy
- Hypoxic encephalopathy/Hypercarbia
- Stroke/Scar epilepsy
- Infection
- Medications

MANAGEMENT

First Aid

- Turn patient to lateral position (preferably left)
- Ensure safe environment
- Give supplemental oxygen
- Assess cause of seizure and consider prognosis, and reversal of underlying cause if consistent with goals of care

Pharmacological

Drug	Stat/Starting Dose	Maintenance Dose
1st line		
Diazepam	PR 10 mg stat May repeat after 5 min	PR 20 mg ON
2nd line		
Midazolam	SC/IV 2.5 to 5 mg stat. Repeat q15 min PRN to abort seizures (up to max of 0.1–0.3 mg/kg)	Start infusion – titrate by SC/IV 0.5 to 1 mg/hr q15 min (up to 0.6 mg/kg/hr) till seizure controlled

(Continued)

Drug	Stat/Starting Dose	Maintenance Dose
3rd line		
Pheno-barbitone	SC 100–200 mg; repeat once after 30 min if necessary, or IV 10–15 mg/kg slow bolus <25 mg/min	SC/IV 0.5–3 mg/kg/day in 1–2 divided doses

- If imminently dying, there is no role for anti-epileptic drugs (AED)
- If consistent with prognosis and goals of care, start AED if no contraindications and AED naïve
- If already on AED, consider increasing AED dose if possibly subtherapeutic +/− reloading if deemed necessary

Drug	Starting Dose	Maintenance Dose
Levetiracetam	PO 750–1000 mg/day in 2 divided doses	1000–3000 mg/day in 2 divided doses; dose adjust in renal failure
Phenytoin	PO/IV 200–300 mg/day or load 10–15 mg/kg slow IV bolus	200–400 mg/day (check serum levels) in single or divided doses
Valproic acid	PO/IV 250–500 mg/day in divided doses	1000–2000 mg/day (check serum levels) in 2–3 divided doses; dose adjust in hepatic failure

Home Care

- There are specific buccal/oromucosal formulations which are currently not available in Singapore
- However, the injection formulations (10mg midazolam hydrochloride) can be administered buccally
- Intranasal administration is not in common use except in the paediatric population

- If continuation of AED is considered necessary when the patient has no PO, SC or IV access, consider NGT if consistent with prognosis and goals of care
- PR route: if on valproic acid or carbamazepine, may switch to rectal preparation or use syrup/suspension rectally; no dose adjustment needed
- Consider admission to hospice or hospital if seizures are refractory

PRACTICAL TIPS

1. The cause of seizures is usually evident in palliative care settings. Further investigations like CT brain and EEG should only be carried out if it significantly alters the management and is consistent with the goals of care.
2. If the patient is going home, teach caregivers about administering rectal diazepam or buccal midazolam.
3. Use levetiracetam (Keppra) in patients with liver impairment.
4. Counsel family caregivers that all medications used to manage seizures can cause sedation. Family members who have witnessed prior seizures often have great fear about seizure recurrence. Review seizure safety with families, including not putting anything in the patient's mouth and making sure the patient is in a safe environment.

REFERENCES

1. Dover Park Hospice MO Orientation Booklet.
2. Droney J, Hall E. Status Epilepticus in a hospice inpatient setting. *J Pain Symptom Manage.* 2008;36(1):97–105.
3. Holsti M, Dudley N, Schunk J, *et al*. Intranasal midazolam vs rectal diazepam for the home treatment of acute seizures in pediatric patients with epilepsy. *Arch Pediatr Adolesc Med.* 2010;164(8):747–753.
4. Tradounsky G. Seizures in palliative care. *Can Fam Physician.* 2013;59(9): 951–955.
5. Kälviäinen R, Reinikainen M. Management of prolonged epileptic seizures and status epilepticus in palliative care patients. *Epilepsy Behav.* 2019; 101(Pt B):106288.

MALIGNANT SPINAL CORD COMPRESSION

Yee Choon Meng

INTRODUCTION

3–5% of patients with cancer have vertebral metastasis. Malignant spinal cord compression (MSCC) occurs in 5 to 10 of every 200 patients with advanced cancer in the last 2 years of their life. The frequency is highest in patients with cancers of the prostate, breast, lung and multiple myeloma. It is important to have a high index of suspicion, as early detection with intervention can help preserve limb function and power.

LEVEL OF SPINE AFFECTED

- Thoracic (60–80%): The least mobile part of the spine
- Lumbosacral (15–20%)
- Cervical (5–10%)

CAUSES

Haematogenous spread with bony metastasis to the vertebra accounts for 85% of MSCC.

The causes include:

- Intramedullary metastasis
- Intradural metastasis
- Extradural compression (80%) due to vertebral body metastasis, causing:
  — Vertebral collapse
  — Tumour spread
  — Interruption of vascular supply (e.g. anterior spinal artery occlusion)

SYMPTOMS AND SIGNS

- Sudden onset of neck pain or back pain/neuropathic band-like pain
- Weakness or numbness in both upper and lower limbs, depending on the level of compression (do a full neurological examination)
- Bowel incontinence/lax anal tone (on per rectal examination)/constipation
- Urinary incontinence/urinary retention/urinary hesitancy
- *Conus Medullaris* — sphincter symptoms and saddle anaesthesia emerge early with mixed upper and lower motor neuron signs (absent ankle jerks and up-going plantars)

TREATMENT

Non-Pharmacological

Surgical

- Surgical decompression (by a spinal surgeon or neurosurgeon)
  — An urgent consult with the spinal surgeon is warranted as this is the only intervention that can salvage neurological function
  — The decision to operate often hinges on the Tokuhashi revised scoring system which includes performance status, the number of extraspinal and vertebral metastasis, the type of cancer and the severity of neurological deficits
  — The Spinal Instability Neoplastic Score (SINS) is a validated tool

to determine clinical spinal instability, used to guide decisions for surgery

Radiotherapy

- Cord compression is an emergency that warrants an urgent referral for radiotherapy
- 20 Gy in five daily fractions or 30 Gy in 10 daily fractions are acceptable regimens
- Single fraction radiotherapy is useful in patients with a very short prognosis
- Patients who undergo surgery followed by adjuvant radiotherapy have better functional outcomes

Pharmacological

- High dose IV/SC/Oral Dexamethasone 16–24 mg/day (i.e. 8–12 mg BD at 8 am/2 pm)
  - While there have been studies supporting an even higher dose of Dexamethasone, it has been associated with a higher incidence of gastrointestinal bleeding and delirium.
- Pain control (Paracetamol/NSAIDs/Opioids)

General Care

- Bowel care
  - Avoid Lactulose as it causes loose acidic stools that precipitate/ worsen bedsores
  - Give Senna or rectal Dulcolax instead
  - Catheterise patient if there is urinary retention
- Physiotherapy/Occupational therapy
- Psychological support for a sudden loss of function
- Caregiver training/nursing care

PRACTICAL TIPS

1. Maintain a high index of suspicion for patients with metastatic disease.
2. Do an early MRI if you suspect cord compression.
   — Make an urgent referral to a spinal surgeon or neurosurgeon (if the patient is a surgical candidate) and/or a radiation oncologist once cord compression is confirmed.

REFERENCES

1. Loblaw DA, Perry J, Chambers A. Systematic review of the diagnosis and management of malignant extradural spinal cord compression: The Cancer Care Ontario Practice Guidelines Initiative's Neurooncology Disease Site Group. *J Clin Oncol.* 2005;23(9):2028–2037.
2. Abrahm J, Banffy M, Harris M. Spinal cord compression in patients with advanced metastatic cancer. *JAMA.* 2008;299(8):937–946.
3. Al-Qurainy EC. Metastatic spinal cord compression: Diagnosis and management. *BMJ* 2016;353:i2539
4. Tokuhashi Y, Matsuzaki H, Oda H, Oshima M, Ryu J. A revised scoring system for preoperative evaluation of metastatic spine tumor prognosis. *Spine (Phila Pa 1976).* 2005;30(19):2186–2191.
5. Patchell RA, Tibbs PA, Regine WF, *et al.* Direct decompressive surgical resection in the treatment of spinal cord compression caused by metastatic cancer: A randomised trial. *Lancet.* 2005;366:643–648.

SUPERIOR VENA CAVA OBSTRUCTION

Lee Chung Seng

INTRODUCTION

Superior vena cava (SVC) syndrome occurs as a result of an obstruction of blood flow through the SVC. The obstruction can be caused by an invasion of, or external compression of the SVC by adjacent structures like the right lung, lymph nodes, other mediastinal structures or by thrombosis of the vessel itself.

CLINICAL FEATURES

Patients may present with dyspnea, facial and upper limb swelling, venous distension in the neck and on the chest wall, dysphagia or stridor and cerebral oedema causing headache, confusion or coma.

A contrast-enhanced thoracic CT would define the level and extent of the venous blockage as well as the underlying cause of the obstruction.

CAUSES

- Lung cancer
- Non-Hodgkin's lymphoma
- Mediastinal Lymphadenopathy: Breast and lung cancers
- Mediastinal tumours: Thymoma, germ cell tumours, mesothelioma

155

- Thrombosis of indwelling central venous catheters
- Post-radiation fibrosis

Intrathoracic malignancy is the most common cause. Lung cancers and Non-Hodgkin's lymphoma account for about 95% of the cases of malignancy-related SVCO.

MANAGEMENT

Non-Pharmacological

- The head should be raised to decrease hydrostatic pressure

Pharmacological

- Dexamethasone 16–24 mg PO/IV should be started on all patients with proven SVCO (It appears to be more useful for steroid-responsive malignancies like lymphoma or patients with thymoma undergoing radiotherapy, particularly those with laryngeal oedema)

Specific Treatment Options

- Chemotherapy for chemo-sensitive tumours like small cell lung cancers, non-Hodgkins lymphoma and germ cell tumours
- Radiotherapy for radiosensitive tumours relieves symptoms within 72 hours and provides complete relief in >60% of lung cancer patients
- Endovascular stenting
- For catheter related thrombosis, remove the catheter and consider anticoagulation

PRACTICAL TIPS

1. There is no additional benefit of one treatment modality over another (radiotherapy, chemotherapy, stenting).
2. However when patients are very symptomatic (dyspneic or stridorous), endovascular stenting is the treatment of choice.

3. Recurrence is about 20% in lung cancer patients who receive chemotherapy and between 10% to 20% in endovascularly stented patients.
4. The IV Cannula should be set on the lower limb (if possible).

REFERENCES

1. Rowell NP, Gleeson FV. Steroids, radiotherapy, chemotherapy and stents for superior vena caval obstruction in carcinoma of bronchus: A systematic review. *Clin Oncol.* 2002;14(5):338–351.
2. Wilson LD, Detterbeck FC. Superior vena cava syndrome with malignant causes. *New Engl J Med.* 2007;356(18):1862–1869.

VENOUS THROMBOEMBOLISM

Ang Ching Ching and Allyn Hum

INTRODUCTION

The spectrum of venous thromboembolism (VTE) is represented by Deep Vein Thrombosis (DVT) and Pulmonary Embolism (PE). It is a common complication in cancer patients who are in a hypercoagulable state. Cancer-associated VTE is often associated with a poor prognosis.

Patients with DVT complain of unilateral swelling of the limbs whereas PE usually presents as dyspnea, pleuritic or substernal chest pain, cough and even syncope and hemoptysis.

CAUSES

The risk factors for cancer associated VTE include:

- Cancer: Haematological, lung, gastrointestinal, brain, kidney, skin, breast, prostate and gynaecological
- Chemotherapy, hormonal and anti-angiogenic therapy
- Central venous catheters

RISK OF CANCER VTE : KHORANA RISK SCORE

Variable	Score
Very high-risk tumor (stomach, pancreas)	2
High-risk tumor (lung, gynecologic, genitourinary excluding prostate)	1
Hemoglobin level <100 g/L or use of red cell growth factors	1
Prechemotherapy leukocyte count >11 × 10⁹/L	1
Prechemotherapy platelet count 350 × 10⁹/L or greater	1
Body mass index 35 kg/m² or greater	1

A score of 0 = low-risk category. A score of 1–2 = intermediate-risk category. A score of >2 = very high-risk category.

INVESTIGATIONS

Normal D-dimer levels likely rule out thromboembolism.

The commonly used confirmatory investigation to confirm DVT is via ultrasound doppler whereas a CT Pulmonary Angiogram (CTPA) or ventilation perfusion (VQ) scan is used for the diagnosis of PE.

MANAGEMENT

Pharmacological

- Low Molecular Weight Heparins (LMWH) given subcutaneously (SC):
  — Enoxaparin (Clexane): 1.5 mg/kg daily or 1 mg/kg q12H
  — Dalteparin (Fragmin): 200 IU/kg for 1 month
                         150 IU/kg daily thereafter
- Direct oral anticoagulants (DOACs):
  — Apixiban : 2.5 mg q12H
  — Rivaroxaban : 10 mg OD
- Warfarin (Vitamin K antagonist):
  — Can be given if LMWH or DOACs are not available
  — Regular blood investigations for dose adjustments, with a chance of drug interactions
  — Target INR: 2.0–3.0

Treatment duration is for at least 6 months in patients with cancer and established VTE to prevent a recurrence.

Treatment beyond 6 months should be considered on an individual basis in patients with active cancer or receiving disease modifying therapy.

Non-Pharmacological

- Inferior Vena Cava Filters (IVC Filters) should not be used as mono-therapy
- IVC filters are used only in these circumstances:
  — Life threatening acute VTE in high risk patients with absolute contraindications to anticoagulant therapy
  — Recurrent embolism while on optimal anticoagulation

PRACTICAL TIPS

1. LMWH and DOACs are currently the drugs of choice in the prevention of cancer associated VTE in high risk patients (Khorana score ≥2) receiving disease modifying treatment.
2. LMWH and DOACs are proven to be more efficacious in the recurrence of cancer associated VTE compared to Warfarin.

REFERENCES

1. Fernandes CJ, Morinaga LTK, Alves JL Jr, *et al*. Cancer-associated thrombosis: The when, how and why. *Eur Respir Rev*. 2019;28:180119
2. Key NS, Khorana AA, Kuderer NM, *et al*. Venous thromboembolism prophy-laxis and treatment in patients with cancer: ASCO clinical practice guideline update. *J Clin Oncol*. 2020;38:5,496–420.
3. Angelini D, Khorana AA. Risk assessment scores for cancer-associated venous thromboembolic disease. *Semin Thromb Hemost*. 2017;43:469–478.

SECTION 6: PSYCHOSOCIAL ISSUES IN PALLIATIVE CARE

ANXIETY

Kwan Yunxin

INTRODUCTION

Significant anxiety symptoms are found in approximately 25% of patients with cancer and they may worsen as the patients become more ill. Anxiety may worsen nausea, vomiting, fatigue, the quality of life and social functioning. It is also common for depression and anxiety to co-exist in palliative care patients.

CAUSES

The common conditions that may cause or precipitate anxiety in palliative care include:

Pain and Dyspnea	—
Hyperactive Delirium	—
Withdrawal Symptoms	Alcohol, Opioids and Benzodiazepines
Drugs	Steroids, Beta-adrenergic agonists
Psychological	Difficulty in coming to terms with cancer, disease progression or failure of treatment

It may be difficult to distinguish the boundaries of normal stress and an anxiety disorder in a patient with advanced illness. A diagnosis of a disorder may be made if the symptoms cause significant distress or significant impairment in the patient's socio-occupational functioning.

COMMON ANXIETY DISORDERS

1. **Generalised Anxiety Disorder**
   - Patients experience excessive anxiety and worry, commonly described as 'free-floating anxiety'. This occurs on more days than not for at least six months, in relation to a number of events or activities that can include financial problems, prognosis or the side-effects of treatment.
   - The patient finds it difficult to control the worry.
   - The anxiety and worry are associated with at least three of the following symptoms: (i) restlessness or feeling tense (ii) being easily fatigued, (iii) difficulty concentrating, (iv) irritability, (v) muscle tension and (vi) sleep disturbance.

2. **Panic Attacks**
   - A panic attack is a sudden, discrete period (or an episode) of intense fear or discomfort that is accompanied by at least four of thirteen symptoms.
   - Symptoms can be somatic or cognitive in nature and include palpitations, sweating, trembling or shaking, sensations of shortness of breath or smothering, feeling of choking, chest pain or discomfort, nausea or abdominal distress, dizziness or light-headedness, derealisation or depersonalisation, fear of losing control or 'going crazy', fear of dying, paresthesias, and chills or hot flushes.
   - There is usually a trigger similar to that for a claustrophobic patient during an MRI (Magnetic Resonance Imaging).

3. **Panic Disorder**
   Recurrent and unexpected panic attacks. At least one of the attacks has been followed by at least one month of one of the following:
   - Persistent concern about having additional attacks.
   - Worry about the implications of the attack or its consequences (e.g. losing control, having a heart attack or losing one's mind).
   - A significant change in behaviour related to the attacks, e.g. needing to be accompanied all the time.

4. **Post-Traumatic Stress Disorder (PTSD)**
   - PTSD is characterised by:
     - i) Re-experiencing an extremely traumatic event (e.g. flashbacks and nightmares);
     - ii) Accompanied by symptoms of increased arousal (e.g. irritability and insomnia); and
     - iii) Avoidance of stimuli associated with the trauma (including places, people and conversations).
   - Patients in palliative care may experience PTSD relating to frightening events associated with their cancer diagnosis or treatment.

APPROACH

- Exclude medical causes, including medications and withdrawal states
- Explore psychological stressors
- Decide on psychological treatments
- Decide on pharmacological treatments

MANAGEMENT

Non-Pharmacological

Psychotherapy

- Patients with mild anxiety may benefit from either supportive or behavioural measures with the goal of increasing the patient's sense of psychological and physical well-being

Psychological interventions include:
- Helping patients to contain the anxiety associated with impending death e.g. frank discussions about patients' fears and anxieties concerning dying have been shown to be effective in alleviating their anxieties
- Assisting patients to manage the practical concerns and fears around the issue of dying, e.g. "Who will take care of my children?"

- Providing information regarding the illness, prognosis and treatment, as well as opportunities for patients to discuss their concerns
- Providing a nurturing and supportive relationship with the patient
- Relaxation skills e.g. deep breathing exercises, progressive muscle relaxation
- Addressing spiritual needs e.g. encouraging patients to speak to their spiritual/religious leaders
- Cognitive Behavioural Therapy
- Support Groups

Pharmacological

- Antidepressants such as Selective Serotonin Reuptake Inhibitors (SSRIs) can also be used to treat anxiety disorders
  — Escitalopram 5–20 mg a day is commonly used as it has fewer interactions with other drugs
- Benzodiazepines have a rapid onset of action and provide quick relief of the patient's anxiety
  — Alprazolam 0.25–1 mg OM-TDS (short-acting, useful for panic attacks)
  — Lorazepam 0.25–1 mg OM-TDS
  — Clonazepam 0.25–1 mg OM-TDS

Lorazepam and Clonazepam are intermediate-acting, and are also useful for generalised anxiety and insomnia.

PRACTICAL TIPS

1. Use Benzodiazepines with caution as they may worsen cognitive impairment or delirium.
2. Short-acting Benzodiazepines with no active metabolites, e.g. Lorazepam, are preferred in patients with impaired hepatic function.
3. Benzodiazepines also cause respiratory depression and interact with opioids and potentiate sedative effects.

REFERENCES

1. Chochinov HM, Breitbart W. Anxiety in palliative care. *Handbook of Psychiatry in Palliative Medicine*, 1ˢᵗ ed. Oxford University Press; 2009, pp. 69–80.
2. Block SD. Psychological issues in end-of-life care. *J Palliat Med.* 2006;9(3): 751–772.

DEPRESSION

Tham Wai Yong and Lim Wen Phei

INTRODUCTION

The prevalence of depression in palliative care patients ranges from 10–42%. The relative risk of depression in cancer exceeds that of stroke, diabetes and heart disease. In oncological and palliative care settings, depression can be debilitating:

- Causes suffering and distress
- Reduces participation in care
- Exacerbates pain and other physical symptoms
- Prolongs length of stay in hospitals
- Impairs treatment adherence
- Associated with poorer prognosis

CAUSES

Depression in palliative care can be attributed to poorly controlled physical symptoms such as pain, nausea and vomiting, as well as psychological reasons such as difficulties in coming to terms with cancer, disease progression or failure of treatment. A history of mental health issues may also predispose patients with life-limiting illnesses to depression.

DIAGNOSING DEPRESSION

Depressive disorders refer to a group of mental health conditions that present primarily with a state of pervasive depressed mood, amongst other symptoms. Patients in palliative care settings may present with clinical symptoms in the spectrum of depressive disorders:

- **Adjustment disorder with depressed mood** refers to a condition that occurs where one has significant difficulties coping with a stressful life event, when a person's usual coping mechanisms are temporarily overwhelmed. It is sometimes informally referred to as "situational depression".
- **Dysthymia (DSM-5: persistent depressive disorder)** is a less severe, but more chronic form of major depression.
- **Major depression** is a mental health condition that is characterised by persistent low mood and/or loss of interest in pleasurable activities, coupled with a variety of cognitive and behavioural symptoms as part of its clinical presentation.

Diagnosing depression in the palliative care setting is challenging. It is particularly challenging to distinguish between the boundaries of normal sadness and depression in the face of life-limiting illness. A major contributing factor to this difficulty is the overlap between somatic and depression symptoms in palliative care. Therefore, the diagnosis hinges on careful examination of the patient's cognition, mood and affect.

Depression is commonly diagnosed using the DSM-5 criteria: ≥5 out of 9 symptoms (including either depressed mood or loss of interest) for more than two weeks. However, some of these symptoms overlap with symptoms present in the medically ill. Endicott (1984) suggested substituting somatic with affective criteria in cancer patients (Table 1).

Table 1: DSM-5 Criteria for Major Depression and Endicott Substitute Symptoms

Symptom	Substitute
• Depressed mood most of the day • Markedly diminished interest or pleasure in all or almost all activities most of the day • Poor appetite or weight changes	Tearfulness or depressed appearance
• Insomnia or hypersomnia • Psychomotor retardation or agitation	Social withdrawal or decreased talkativeness
• Fatigue or loss of energy	Brooding, self-pity or pessimism
• Diminished ability to think or concentrate, indecisiveness • Suicidal ideation	Lack of reactivity; cannot be cheered up

MANAGEMENT

- Treat physical symptoms and exclude delirium; note that both conditions can exist concurrently
- Consider acutely demoralising factors and address situational reactions by supporting patients dealing with acute stressors
- Introduce psychological interventions as appropriate to the patient's needs, personhood and agreement to psychotherapeutic treatment
- Psychosocial interventions as part of early palliative care can reduce later-life distress and adverse impact on quality of life
- Consider pharmacological therapy for patients with significant and persistent symptoms

Psychosocial Interventions

Psychotherapeutic interventions are essential in the management of psychological distress and depressive symptoms at the end of life. They may complement and enhance the effectiveness of pharmacological treatments. Furthermore, pharmacological options are often limited at the end of life.

Supportive Psychotherapy	• Includes active listening and supportive verbal interventions
Hypnotherapy	• Useful in anxiety, sleep difficulties, modifying pain and other symptoms
Narrative Therapy	• Creation of a 'legacy document', celebrating the life of the individual
Dignity Therapy	• Provides a framework and questions to guide the goals of care and interventions that have dying with dignity as a targeted outcome
Relaxation-Guided Imagery	• Reduces anxiety and improves coping
Cognitive-Behavioural Therapy	• Reduces symptoms of physical and emotional distress, promotes active coping strategies; targets dysfunctional cognitions concerning disease and symptoms
Meaning-Centred Therapy	• Targets hopelessness and a desire for hastened death
Creative Arts Therapy	• Music and art therapy may reduce pain, fatigue, depression and anxiety in oncological and palliative care settings • Good option for patients who are not verbally expressive, or experience demoralisation from prolonged hospitalisation

PHARMACOLOGICAL

There are several classes of antidepressants available. Antidepressants are effective, not addictive, and do not lose their efficacy over time. General principles to consider when prescribing antidepressants in palliative care settings include:

- Drug-drug interactions (e.g. opioids, chemotherapeutic agents)
- Onset of action
- Tolerability of possible side effects
- Switch treatments early (1–2 weeks) if there are intolerable side effects, or if no improvement at all is observed despite therapeutic doses (3–4 weeks)

In palliative care, Escitalopram (it has a more rapid onset of two weeks and better side-effect profile), as well as Mirtazapine (a rapid onset, nocturnal sedation and appetite-stimulating effect), are commonly used.

- Selective Serotonin Reuptake Inhibitors (SSRIs)
  — Escitalopram 5–20 mg ON (least pharmacokinetic interactions)
  — Fluoxetine 20 mg OM/Fluvoxamine 50 mg ON/Sertraline 50 mg OM (may take 6 weeks to take effect)
  — As a group, they can cause nausea and the syndrome of inappropriate anti-diuretic hormone secretion (SIADH)
- Noradrenergic and Specific Serotonergic Antidepressant (NaSSA)
  — Mirtazapine 7.5–30 mg ON (can be used sublingually as a soluble tablet)
  — Can be sedating, an advantage in patients with insomnia
- Tricyclic Antidepressants (TCA)
  — Amitriptyline 25–150 mg ON, Nortriptyline 25–150 mg ON
  — Can be used as a neuropathic pain adjuvant but can cause arrhythmias and anticholinergic side-effects
  — Avoid in the elderly
- Serotonin Norepinephrine Reuptake Inhibitor (SNRI)
  — Venlafaxine 37.5–225 mg OM
  — Duloxetine 30–60 mg OM (useful as neuropathic pain adjuvant)
  — Can cause hypertension and tachycardia due to noradrenergic effects
- Norepinephrine Dopamine Reuptake Inhibitor
  — Bupropion 75–300 mg OM
  — Can be stimulating and lower seizure threshold

- Serotonin modulators:
  - Trazodone 50–100 mg ON
  - May cause sedation, often used in insomnia, or used off-label in patients with behavioural and psychological symptoms of dementia
- Psychostimulants
  - Methylphenidate 2.5–10 mg 4–6 hourly (avoid in the evening as can cause insomnia)
  - An option in significantly fatigued patients who do not respond adequately to antidepressants
  - Can cause tachycardia, hypertension, nausea and lowers seizure threshold
  - Use at low doses and with caution in the elderly

PRACTICAL TIPS

1. All palliative care providers can provide good psychosocial and mental health care.
2. Understanding the patient's personhood, coping mechanisms and worldview as experienced before the onset of depression helps discern the difference between normal sadness and depression.
3. Often, several sessions are required to observe and elicit depressive symptoms.
4. The choice of antidepressants depends on the onset of action, side-effect profile, cost and its usefulness as a pain adjuvant.
5. Methylphenidate and Bupropion are useful for patients with apathetic depression.
6. When using atypical antidepressants, consider continued access to medications (financial support for non-standard medications, availability of medications in drug formulary of the receiving care provider) should the patient be discharged to the community.
7. Family therapy sessions may be useful when there are complicated family dynamics.
8. There is also a growing body of evidence for the importance of enquiring for, and addressing the spiritual needs of patients with advanced life-limiting illnesses.

REFERENCES

1. Mitchell AJ, Chan M, Bhatti H, Halton M, Grassi L, Johansen C, Meader N. Prevalence of depression, anxiety, and adjustment disorder in oncological, haematological, and palliative-care settings: A meta-analysis of 94 interview-based studies. *Lancet Oncol*. 2011 Feb 1;12(2):160–174.
2. Rayner L, Price A. Antidepressants for the treatment of depression in palliative care: Systematic review and meta-analysis. *Palliat Med*. 2011;25(1):36–51.

GRIEF AND BEREAVEMENT

Kwan Yunxin

INTRODUCTION

The loss of a loved one ushers in a period of intense emotional distress, which may be viewed as unusual and distressing. Both clinicians and bereaved individuals worry about whether the experience is normal.

NORMAL GRIEF

Initial grief often manifests as a 'state of shock' that may be expressed as a feeling of numbness. Despite the denial and protest, emotions such as pining and yearning are also experienced.

As death is comprehended, the bereaved individual experiences a 'state of acute and intense anguish'. This may be accompanied by feelings of guilt and anger, preoccupation with thoughts of the deceased and social withdrawal.

'Resolution' gradually takes place as full knowledge of the loss is cognitively and emotionally integrated. The bereaved individual is able to resume old roles like returning to work, acquire new roles, experience pleasure without guilt, and seek the companionship and love of others.

The expression of grief varies from person to person as it depends on cultural norms and expectations. Generally, normal grief causes only mild and transient functional impairment and improves with time.

COMPLICATED GRIEF

Complicated grief which results from the failure of transition from acute to integrated grief occurs in about 10% of bereaved individuals. The grief may be prolonged, overly intense, delayed or absent.

Characteristics of complicated grief include:

- Guilt about things other than actions taken or not taken by the survivor at the time of the death
- Suicidal ideas
- Morbid preoccupation with worthlessness
- Excessive preoccupation with the deceased
- Marked psychomotor retardation
- Prolonged and marked functional impairment
- Hallucinatory experiences other than thinking that he or she hears the voice of or transiently sees the image of the deceased person

Risk factors for complicated grief are:

- Sudden, unexpected, untimely death
- Especially close or ambivalent relationship with the deceased
- History of mood or anxiety disorders
- History of multiple important losses or adverse life events
- Poor health
- Concurrent stressors
- Lack of social support

It is important to assess for depression and anxiety disorders during bereavement. Bereaved individuals are also vulnerable to a decline in general medical health, including cardiovascular disease and poor self-care.

MANAGEMENT

Non-Pharmacological

- Most bereaved individuals do not require professional intervention

- Practical help, a listening ear and reassurance that their grief is normal may be all the bereaved individual requires

Pharmacological

- Lorazepam 0.5 mg ON PRN (low dose Benzodiazepines) can be used to relieve persistent insomnia (<2 weeks)
- Fluvoxamine 50 mg ON (Anti-depressants) may be used in complicated grief, depression or anxiety disorders

PRACTICAL TIPS

1. It is important to ensure that the patient's loved ones do not neglect their own health and needs.
2. Moderate or severe functional impairment is a good indicator of complicated grief.
3. We grieve for our patients who have passed on as well. Helping the bereaved loved ones of our patients may remind us of our own experiences with grief, which may enhance or interfere with our ability to help. Speaking to our colleagues or supervisors will be helpful in facing our difficulties.

REFERENCES

1. Zisook S, Shear K. Grief and bereavement: What psychiatrists need to know. *World Psychiatry*. 2009;8(2):67–74
2. Practical death-related matters: https://www.nea.gov.sg/our-services/after-death/post-death-matters
3. Grief counselling providers: https://singaporehospice.org.sg/community-bereavement-service-providers/

SPIRITUAL CARE

Tricia Yung

INTRODUCTION

Patients with advanced, life-limiting illnesses may experience spiritual distress as they try to find meaning and purpose in the midst of suffering. This important dimension of suffering must be addressed as it will heighten physical, emotional and social distress.

Spirituality is a broad term that has no universally accepted definition. Some suggestions include:

- The way individuals seek and express meaning and purpose, and the way they experience their connectedness to the moment, to self, to others, to nature, and to the significant or sacred
- About what we do with our unrest, desire, anxiety, longings and pain
- Integration of different parts of the self, thereby experiencing healing, growth, and connection with self, others, God and the universe

EXISTENTIAL SUFFERING

Serious illness often triggers questions of a spiritual nature—questions of meaning, value, and relationships. Common spiritual concerns include "Is God punishing me?", "What is the meaning of my life?". Patients often encounter feelings of:

• Anxiety	• Loss of personal meaning
• Fear of being a burden	• Loss of purpose in life
• Fear of death	• Loss of dignity
• Hopelessness	• Loneliness

SPIRITUAL HISTORY

Goals in a spiritual history include:

- Learning (and sharing as appropriate) about spiritual and religious beliefs
- Assessing level of spiritual distress or helping them draw upon their strengths
- Providing compassionate care
- Assisting with finding inner resources for healing and acceptance
- Determining spiritual/religious beliefs that could affect treatment choices
- Identifying the need for a referral to a trained medical social worker, chaplain or other spiritual care provider

SPIRITUAL ASSESSMENT TOOLS

Several spiritual assessment tools (represented by their mnemonics) have been used primarily in the clinical setting for non-chaplain clinicians to efficiently integrate open-ended questions into a standard medical history.

These include:

Tools	Examples
FICA Faith and Belief	Do you have spiritual beliefs that help you cope with stress? What gives your life meaning?
Importance	Have your beliefs influenced how you take care of yourself in this illness?

(Continued)

Tools	Examples
Community Address	Are you part of a spiritual or religious community? Is this of support to you and how? How would you like me to address these issues in your health care?
HOPE Source of Hope, meaning and comfort Organized religion Personal spirituality/ practices Effects on care	What are your sources of hope or comfort ? What helps you during difficult times? Are you a member of an organized religion? What religious practices are important to you? Do you have spiritual beliefs that are separate from religion? What spiritual practices are most helpful to you? Is there any conflict between your beliefs and the care you will be receiving? Do you hold beliefs or follow practices that you believe may affect your care?
SPIRIT Spiritual belief Personal spirituality Integration with spiritual community Ritualized practices And restrictions	What is your religious affiliation? Describe your religious belief system. Describe the beliefs and practices of your religion or spiritual system. What does your spirituality/religion mean to you? What is the importance of your spirituality/religion in daily life? Do you belong to any spiritual or religious group or community? What importance does this group have for you? Is it a source of support? Are there specific practices that you carry out/or forbid as part of your religion/spirituality?

(Continued)

(Continued)

Tools	Examples
Implications for medical care Terminal event planning	What aspects of your religion/spirituality would you like me to keep in mind as I care for you? As we plan for your care near the end of life, how does your faith affect your decisions?

PRACTICAL TIPS

1. Focus on the process (the process of searching for meaning and saying it's OK not to know now and not to have a solution).
2. Consider asking these specific questions about spirituality if you have limited time:
   a) Are you at peace?
   b) What gives you your sense of meaning and purpose?
   c) What really matters to you in your life?
3. Allow empathic listening and use questions that promote reflection to create space for the patient to make connections and changes.
4. Help the patient to connect with what goes on beyond the layers of behaviour/struggle. Help the patient to live with the questions. Eg. What is this struggle saying to you? Where do you find your peace even when there is no answer?
5. Focus on the healing of the whole person and growth rather than the solution to problems; being at peace with oneself.
6. Respect the patient's religious and spiritual experiences for healing.
7. Refer to medical social workers, pastoral care or chaplains for further advice and support.

REFERENCES

1. National Consensus Conference in US. Guidelines for Interprofessional Clinical Spiritual Care 2009.
2. Puchalski C, Ferrell B, Virani R, *et al.* Improving the quality of spiritual care as a dimension of palliative care: the report of the Consensus Conference. *J Palliat Med.* 2009;(10):885–904.

3. Puchalski C, Romer AL. Taking a spiritual history allows clinicians to understand patients more fully. *J Palliat Med.* 2000;3(1):129–137.

4. Anandarajah G, Hight E. Spirituality and medical practice: using the HOPE questions as a practical tool for spiritual assessment. *Am Fam Physician.* 2001;63(1):81–89.

5. Maugans TA. The SPIRITual history. *Arch Fam Med.* 1996;5(1):11–16.

6. Steinhauser KE, Voils CI, Clipp EC, Bosworth HB, Christakis NA, Tulsky JA. "Are you at peace?": one item to probe spiritual concerns at the end of life. *Arch Intern Med.* 2006;166(1):101–105.

SECTION 7: COMMUNICATION

BREAKING BAD NEWS

Lynn Wiryasaputra and Mervyn Koh

INTRODUCTION

Breaking bad news to your patient and their loved ones is an integral part of every clinician's job. It usually involves the disclosure of an incurable or life-altering illness, or the news that your patient is dying.

Bad news is not just restricted to life-limiting issues – information about becoming dependent on a mobility aid or the need for diet texture modification may also have adverse consequences on a patient's overall well-being.

THE SPIKES PROTOCOL

A recommended and commonly used method is the 6-part SPIKES Protocol conceived by Buckman et al.

Setting

- Familiarise yourself with the patient's medical history.
- Ensure that individuals who are important to the patient are invited to join the family meeting.
- Find a quiet and comfortable room with seats for everyone – switch your mobile phone to silent mode.
- Be punctual.
- Introduce everyone in the medical team.

191

Perception

- Ask your patient about his/her understanding of their medical condition "What do you understand about your medical condition so far?" or "What has your doctor told you about your illness?"

Invitation

- Extend an invitation to your patient to see how much they would like to know: "Would you like to know more about your illness/the results of the CT scan?"
- Give a warning shot and allow your patient to opt out: "I am afraid the results are not good. Would you still like me to continue?"

Knowledge

- If your patient agrees, give the news in a clear and exact manner: "The scan shows that there is a growth in the lung. This is most likely due to lung cancer."
- Pitch the complexity of information delivered at an appropriate level for your patient.
- Check back to ensure that your patient accurately understands the information you have given.
- Give your patient the opportunity to ask questions.

Empathize: NURSE Your Patient's Emotions

- Be sensitive to your patient's emotions and non-verbal cues *throughout the family meeting* – <u>Name</u> the emotion as it helps your patient feel validated.
- Get a deeper <u>understanding</u> of why your patient is feeling that way: Be mindful of what they are thinking/feeling through the questions they may ask you.
- Respond <u>Respectfully</u> to the expressed emotion of your patient and their loved ones.
  - → Avoid trivialising your patient's concerns: "Don't worry about the side effects of chemotherapy."

→ Be comfortable with silence and tears. Allow them the time to talk, cry or be silent. Do not be in a hurry to comfort them.

→ Don't ignore questions you cannot answer. If you're uncertain about something, seek clarification from a senior doctor.

- <u>Support</u> your patient as they are still absorbing the shock of the news. This can be done with your words and actions: "I will come by to see you again to ensure that your nausea and vomiting is well controlled."

A common pitfall is that clinicians only offer a sprinkling of Empathic statements towards the end of a family meeting! Proactively train and tune your 'emotional radar' to be sensitive to the psycho-emotional needs of your patient.

Strategy and Summary

- Have a clear plan of action.
- Summarise the information already given in a short and succinct manner.

PRACTICAL TIPS

1. These are some 'empathic phrases' which may be useful when communicating bad news to patients/families:

   "This news must be very upsetting for you."
   "This must be difficult for you."

2. Say it only if you mean it, otherwise it will fall flat.

REFERENCES

1. Baile W, Buckman R, Lenzi R. SPIKES — A 6-step protocol for delivering bad news: Application to the patient with cancer. *Oncologist*. 2000;5: 302–311.
2. Back A, Arnold R, Baile W, Tulsky J. Approaching difficult communication tasks in oncology. *CA Cancer J Clinicians*. 2005;55:164–167.
3. Hum A, Koh M. *The Bedside Communication Handbook: Speaking with Patients and Families*. Singapore: World Scientific Publishing; 2021.

GOALS OF CARE DISCUSSIONS

Lynn Wiryasaputra and Mervyn Koh

INTRODUCTION

Establishing the goals of care for your patient is imperative in ensuring that quality care can be delivered, according to your patient's preferences. These conversations should be carried out especially when patients are at risk of sudden demise or when patients with life-limiting illnesses are in an acute hospital setting.

We should no longer reserve these conversations to the end of life. Having these conversations earlier leads to better quality of life, reduced use of non-beneficial medical care near death, positive family outcomes, and reduced costs.

'GOALS OF CARE' OPTIONS

These decisions can usually be classified under the following main categories:

a. ICU Care: Use of CPR/intubation
b. General Ward Care: Use of fluid resuscitation, inotropes, antibiotics and blood transfusions at the medical team's discretion
c. Comfort Measures: Keeping the patient comfortable

Address the Issue of Cardio-Pulmonary Resuscitation

- Some families may not understand that in certain instances, CPR will not be performed due to its futility. This needs to be clearly explained to them beforehand to prevent misunderstandings.

  Here are some practical guidelines for junior clinicians who are often tasked to lead these challenging and emotionally charged discussions:

Have a Plan in Mind

- The senior doctor of the team (consultant/registrar) should make a recommendation as to the 'extent' of care which suits the patient best.

Do Not 'Offer a Menu'

- Never offer the patient/family a 'menu' of choices as to 'how to proceed'.
- Doing this unfairly delegates the medical decision-making process to the families who often do not have the knowledge and are not in the best position to decide for the patient.
- This may lead to the inappropriate choice of aggressive treatment which may not be in the best interests of the patient at that time.

Remind Them of What Has Been Done and What Will Be Done for the Patient

- Revisit the previous treatment which was given to your patient and explain why the treatment did not work/why your patient is no longer a suitable candidate for that treatment.
- Ensure that they do not feel abandoned – emphasize that the medical team will still give the necessary medication to keep the patient's symptoms controlled.
  - This is to reassure them that the patient is not being neglected just because a less aggressive treatment is recommended.

REFERENCES

1. Quill T. Initiating end-of-life discussions with seriously ill patients; Addressing the 'Elephant in the Room'. *JAMA*. 2000;284(19):2502–2507.
2. Bernacki R. Block S. Communication about serious illness care goals: A review and synthesis of best practices. *JAMA Intern Med*. 2013;174(12): 1994–2003.

ADVANCE CARE PLANNING

Raymond Ng

Advance Care Planning (ACP) is a process whereby patients discuss, state and document their values and wishes regarding medical care with their caregivers, in the event that they are incapacitated from making decisions on their own. ACP explores that which is important to individuals, helps to honour their preferences with regard to treatment near the end of life and decreases the caregiver's burden in decision-making.

ACP and the AMD

In Singapore, the Advance Medical Directive (AMD) is a legal process enabling patients to state in advance their preference not to receive extraordinary life-sustaining treatment in the event that they become incapable of making decisions and are suffering from terminal illness. The AMD is one part of the broader concept of ACP.

Suggested Interview Template (Adapted from *Respecting Choices®*)

1. **Assess the motivation, knowledge and beliefs of the individual you are assisting**
    *   "What do you understand about advance care planning and/or advanced directives?"

2. **Explore the understanding of health/medical condition**
   - "Can you tell me what you understand about your condition."
   - "How has your health condition changed in the past few months?"
   - "It seems you have questions about your health condition. We should write these down for you to discuss with your physician/nurse/other healthcare provider."
   (Provide information only if the facilitator is able to do so or where appropriate).
3. **Explore experiences**
   - "Have you had experiences with family or friends who became seriously ill and decisions were made about life-sustaining treatment?"
   - "What did you learn from those experiences?"
   - "I see that you were in the hospital recently. What did that experience mean to you, if anything?"
4. **Explore the concept of 'living well'**
   - "What activities or experiences are most important for you to live well?" or "What gives your life meaning?"
   - "What fears or worries do you have about your illness or medical care?" or "What needs or services would you like to discuss?"
   - "What helps you when you face serious challenges in life?" or "Do you have religious or spiritual beliefs that are important to you?"
5. **Explore the understanding of potential complications with patient/resident or healthcare agent**
   - "As you know, you have an illness that makes it difficult to predict when a complication may occur and decisions may have to be made on your behalf. Do you know what complications may occur? These conditions may be life limiting."
   (Provide information only if the facilitator is able to do so or where appropriate).
6. **Help make informed treatment decisions**
   - "There are decisions you may need to make. These include considering whether or not to receive nutrition, fluids, hospitalisation, surgery or comfort care. We want you to learn more and have time to think about the goals and the preferences you may have."

- Regarding CPR:
  - i) Explore the understanding of CPR
    - "What do you understand about CPR? What has your physician told you about CPR?"
  - ii) Explore the understanding of benefits and burdens of CPR, and provide information as appropriate
    - "What do you know about the success of CPR? CPR is not as successful as you think."
  - iii) Explore the goals for treatment
    - "What outcome would you expect from CPR? What would be an unacceptable outcome?"
  - iv) Explore fears and concerns
    - "Do you have any fears or concerns about making this decision?"
    - Explain other options where appropriate e.g. artificial ventilation.

7. **Develop a list of questions or concerns and involve others where necessary**
   - Encourage the individual to involve others who can address their concerns and/or provide information.
   - Draw up a list of questions for the appropriate person to address.

8. **Explore the individual's perspective of comfort care**
   - "There are many things we can do to make you comfortable. Can you tell me what being comfortable means to you? What fears or concerns do you have?

PRACTICAL TIPS

Guide for Healthcare Professionals on Communication During ACP

1. Ensure that you have been appropriately trained to discuss ACP, have rapport with the individual and have adequate knowledge of the individual and potential treatment options.
2. ACP should be voluntary.
3. Ensure that the discussion is held in a comfortable and unhurried setting.

4. Ask open-ended questions.
5. Give information in ways the individual understands. Check that you have understood the individual correctly and summarise at the end of the discussion.
6. Remember to foster the person's agenda. Endeavour to maintain trust and rapport throughout the conversation. Understand the basis of the person's decisions.
7. Be self-aware, non-judgemental and do not impose one's values on the process of ACP facilitation.
8. Reassure the individual that their decisions can be re-visited at any time and changed. ACP is not a single event but an on-going process with periodic reviews where appropriate.
9. Acknowledge and respect the individual's culture, religion and beliefs.
10. It is prudent to check if the person would like to have their loved ones present when having the conversation, especially the person whom they would like to nominate as the healthcare spokesperson.
11. Document the statement of wishes and date all subsequent changes. Ensure that the information is shared with the medical teams managing the patient in all settings of care.

REFERENCES

1. The Advanced Medical Directive. Ministry of Health, Singapore. https://www.moh.gov.sg/policies-and-legislation/advance-medical-directive. Accessed 12/10/2020.
2. Hum A, Koh M. *The Bedside Communication Handbook: Speaking with Patients and Families*. Singapore: World Scientific Publishing; 2021.

AN APPROACH TO ETHICAL CASE ANALYSIS IN PALLIATIVE CARE

Neo Han Yee

Management of patients with advanced illnesses frequently involves value-laden discussions on perceived quality-of-life, burden of treatment and medical futility. These discussions may carry medico-legal implications, the mitigation of which will require physicians to be familiar with local ethical guidelines and relevant healthcare laws. A structured approach to such ethically-complex issues will help give clarity.

Step 1 — Define the Ethical Problem as A Concise Question

Define the issues and associated conflicting ethical principles using 2–3 concise sentences. This exercise compels the clinician to distil concerns into tangible problem statements that can then be specifically addressed. Examples of common ethical questions include:

- Does Mr ABC possess mental capacity to refuse life-saving amputation of his gangrenous foot?
- Can the son of Mr DEF demand continuation of extraordinary life-sustaining treatment when further treatment is no longer deemed clinically beneficial by the ICU physician?

- Can spinal surgery be performed on a migrant worker presenting with acute spinal cord compression against the wishes of his employer who is legally obligated to pay for his treatment?

Step 2 — Compartmentalize Relevant Information Using Jonsen's 4 Boxes

A 4-box tool kit was developed by Jonsen et al to help clinicians collate information pertinent to formulating a measured decision. Figure 1 summarizes common information that clinicians need to gather, grouped into the four domains of (i) Clinical Indication, (ii) Patient Preferences, (iii) Quality-of-Life and (iv) Contextual Features. Beginners are encouraged to move through the quadrants in the following order:

- **Clinical Indication.** This will include information on disease severity, reversibility, prognosis and treatment options. Consideration will also have to be given to the benefit and burden of treatment options, as well as the implications of non-treatment.
- **Patient Preference.** A valid consent (or refusal) of treatment comprises of (i) adequate mental capacity; (ii) disclosure of material information; and (iii) freedom from coercive influence. Clinicians will need to evaluate the patient's ability to understand, appreciate, retain and weigh the information encapsulated in the first quadrant, as well as empower patients to express their decision in a clear and comprehensible manner.
- **Quality-of-Life.** As far as possible, judgment on quality-of-life should be based on a mentally competent patient's subjective perception. If the patient has lost mental capacity, consideration should be given to their previously expressed values. Objective parameters such as best anticipated physical (ability to self-care) and cognitive functions should also be factored into this deliberation.
- **Contextual Features.** This quadrant comprises multiple domains including:
  - Healthcare Legislations and Case Laws e.g. Mental Capacity Act, Advanced Medical Directive Act, Employment of Foreign Manpower Act, Vulnerable Adult Act, Modified Montgomery Test, Bolam's Test and the Bolitho Addendum.

MEDICAL INDICATIONS	PATIENT PREFERENCES
Beneficence and Nonmaleficence • What is the patient's medical problem? History? Diagnosis? Prognosis? • Is the problem acute? Chronic? Critical? Emergent? Reversible? • What are the goals of treatment? • What are the probabilities of success? • What are the plans in case of therapeutic failure? • In sum, how can this patient be benefited by medical and nursing care, and how can harm be avoided?	**Respect for Patient Autonomy** • Is the patient mentally capable and legally competent? Is there evidence of capacity? • If competent, what is the patient stating about preferences for treatment? • Has the patient been informed of benefits and risks, understood this information, and given consent? • If incapacitated, who is the appropriate surrogate? Is the surrogate using appropriate standards for decision making? • Has the patient expressed prior preferences (eg, advance directives)? • Is the patient unwilling or unable to cooperate with medical treatment? If so, why? • In sum, is the patient's right to choose being respected to the extent possible in ethics and law?
QUALITY OF LIFE	**CONTEXTUAL FEATURES**
Beneficence, Nonmaleficence, and Respect for Patient Autonomy • What are the prospects, with or without treatment, for a return to normal life? • What physical, mental, and social deficits is the patient likely to experience if treatment succeeds? • Are there biases that might prejudice the provider's evaluation of the patient's quality of life? • Is the patient's present or future condition such that his or her continued life might be judged as undesirable? • Is there any plan and rationale to forgo treatment? • Are there plans for comfort and palliative care?	**Loyalty and Fairness** • Are there family issues that might influence treatment decisions? • Are there provider (physician, nurse) issues that might influence treatment decisions? • Are there financial and economic factors? • Are there religious or cultural factors? • Are there limits on confidentiality? • Are there problems of allocation of resources? • How does the law affect treatment decisions? • Is clinical research or teaching involved? • Is there any conflict of interest on the part of the providers or the institution?

Fig. 1:   Jonsen's 4-Topics Approach

Schumann JH, Alfandre D. Clinical ethical decision making: the four topics approach. Semin Med Pract. 2008;11:36–42.

— Religious Beliefs and Cultural Convictions.

— Equitable Resource Allocation e.g. rationing policies concerning allocation of scarce resources.

— Social Vulnerability and Financial concerns that may influence management decisions.

Step 3 — Weighing Conflicting Ethical Principles

The 4-box approach does not in itself resolve any ethical conundrums. However, it serves the purpose of anchoring facts to principles, thereby enabling the clinicians to appreciate what is ethically relevant. For the clinician to formulate an ethically defensible plan, he will need to identify and weigh conflicting ethical principles (Beneficence, Non-Maleficence, Autonomy and Social Justice), plotting a course of action best befitting the patient's overall best interests, as well as their expressed wishes against professional and legal regulations.

REFERENCE

1.   Jonsen A, Siegler M, Winslade W. Clinical ethics: A practical approach to ethical decisions in clinical medicine, 7th ed. New York, NY: McGraw-Hill; 2010.

SECTION 8: COMMUNITY SERVICES

COMMUNITY PALLIATIVE CARE SERVICES

Chia Gerk Sin

Palliative care extends from acute healthcare settings into the community. To achieve a smooth transition of care, it is important to understand the scope of these palliative community services in order to communicate how they can lend support to patients and their families. Palliative community services complement tertiary inpatient care, hospice home care and hospice day care.

INPATIENT HOSPICE PALLIATIVE CARE SERVICES (IHPCS)

IHPCS are institutions where general palliative and/or specialised palliative care can be provided. These institutions are either inpatient hospices or palliative care wards within selected community hospitals. Admissions can be covered by Medishield and Medisave.

Inpatient Hospices

Most inpatient hospices in Singapore provide both general and specialised palliative care. They have a multi-disciplinary team of nurses, doctors and therapists who provide holistic care addressing the physical, psychological, social and spiritual well-being of an individual. Inpatient hospices typically admit patients with life-limiting illnesses with a prognosis of less than three months. On an individual basis, inpatient hospices will also care for patients with advanced illnesses based on needs, even if the prognosis is estimated at more than 3 months.

The philosophy of inpatient hospice care is to enhance quality of life, with the focus on optimising the management of symptoms like pain, dyspnoea and delirium, ensuring that patients are comfortable at the end of life. Hospices also offer music and art therapy, palliative rehabilitation as well as spiritual care.

There are presently, three inpatient hospices in Singapore, located at different parts of the island, all of which are accessible by public transport. They are Dover Park Hospice, Assisi Hospice and St Joseph's Home.

Palliative Care wards in Community Hospital (CH)

These are transitional care sites for patients with palliative care needs awaiting:

1. Completion of intravenous treatment e.g. prolonged course of antibiotics for complicated infections
2. Arrival of a domestic helper to continue care at home
3. Completion of caregiving training
4. Care of complex wounds

Patients who are accepted into the palliative wards in CH usually have discharge plans finalised in the acute hospital prior to transfer of care. During the course of stay in the CH, the team may engage the patients and their families in Advance Care Planning (ACP) if this has not already been done in the acute care hospital.

Community hospitals with palliative wards include St Andrew's, SingHealth Community Hospitals and St Luke's Hospital amongst others.

HOME HOSPICE SERVICES

Home hospice services support patients with advanced cancer or non-cancer illnesses who have a prognosis of less than 12 months. The service is anchored by nurses, with medical support from doctors, psychosocial support by medical social workers (MSW) and art/music therapists in the familiarity of the patient's home. The team empowers families and caregivers to provide good care for their loved ones at the end of life through caregiver training, phone consults and pre-arranged physical visits at home.

Visits are scheduled by the nurses on a "as needed" basis to address new or worsening symptoms or to follow up after discharge from the hospital. Besides access to the homecare team during office hours, the patient and family can also receive advice in the event of a crisis through a hotline number which is operational outside of office hours and on weekends and public holidays.

Hospice home care teams have the expertise and experience to support the care of terminally ill patients who wish to spend their last days in their own homes, including the initiation of infusions at home to alleviate suffering at the end of life. The MSW and therapists are also involved to support families through this difficult period of bereavement. Many times, bereavement support will continue beyond the period of the patient's demise if needed.

To facilitate the smooth transition of care and empower our community partners in the care for patients in their homes, we will need to remember the following points:

1. Proper handover of patient's care

   - Detailed discharge summaries with essential issues that arose during admission faxed or emailed to the relevant team
   - Phone handover of pertinent issues that cannot be adequately addressed in the discharge summaries to the homecare nurse in charge

2. **Explaining the role of the hospice home care team to patients and families**

    The hospice home care team is a consultative service caring for patients with a prognosis of less than 12 months. The team specialises in managing symptoms that arise from complications of the advanced illness in the patient's own home. Care and change of medical devices (i.e. Indwelling urine catheter, Nasogastric tubes) may also be undertaken by the hospice home care team but may be redirected to other home nursing teams in exceptional circumstances.

    The list of hospice home care service providers include:

Assisi Hospice	Metta Hospice Care
Buddhist Compassion Relief Tzu-Chi Foundation (Singapore)	Methodist Welfare Services
Dover Park Hospice	Singapore Cancer Society
HCA Hospice Care	Tsao Foundation (Hua Mei Mobile Clinic)

HOSPICE DAY CARE

The objective of hospice day care is to allow social engagement amongst patients who have advanced illnesses, allowing them to live life to the fullest by making each day count. Hospice day care engagement includes singing sessions, art making, light group exercises, chit-chatting sessions with fellow day care attendees and excursions out and about Singapore.

The hospice day care centre is managed by a team of nurses, doctors, therapists and committed volunteers. Participants can arrange to attend day care at a frequency ranging from several times a week to daily depending on their social circumstances. Hospice day care centres operate on weekdays, except public holidays from mid-morning to late afternoon. Meals as well as two-way transportation is provided.

Hospice Day Care requirements:

1. Patients need to have good sitting tolerance and stamina as they will be seated on cushioned recliners or wheelchairs

2. Caregivers need to be able to:
   (a) Bring patients to the pick-up point
   (b) Fetch the patient home from the drop off point
3. If the patient requires oxygen, please contact the respective centre to check as there are facility constraints that would limit the number of patients accepted
4. Laboratory services are not available

List of Hospice Day Care Centres:

1. Assisi Hospice
2. Dover Park Hospice
3. HCA Hospice Care

REFERENCES

1. Singapore Hospice Council Website, www.singaporehospice.org.sg
2. Haukland EC, von Plessen C, Nieder C, *et al.* Adverse events in deceased hospitalised cancer patients as a measure of quality and safety in end-of-life cancer care. *BMC Palliat Care.* 2020;19:76. https://doi.org/10.1186/s12904-020-00579-0

SECTION 9: OPIOIDS AND ADJUVANT ANALGESICS

CODEINE

Chia Siew Chin

WHAT IS CODEINE?

Codeine is a weak opioid, with about one-tenth the potency of Morphine. It is metabolised to Codeine-6-glucuronide (80%) and Morphine via the CYP2D6 enzymes. The active metabolites are excreted via the kidneys.

Most of the analgesic effect comes from the metabolism into Morphine. There is a large variation between different individuals in the metabolism to Morphine. Poor metabolisers produce little or no Morphine and thus experience little analgesic effect; ultra-rapid metabolisers produce greater than normal amounts of Morphine, which can lead to opioid toxicity.

WHAT ARE THE AVAILABLE FORMULATIONS?

- Codeine may come in the form of:
  - Codeine tablets — 30 mg
  - Panadeine (combined with paracetamol) which contains 500 mg of paracetamol and 8 mg of Codeine
  - Linctus for cough
- Onset of action: 30–60 minutes
- Duration of action: 4–6 hours

WHEN DO WE USE CODEINE?

It is used mainly in mild to moderate pain. It is not as commonly used due to the interindividual variation in metabolism, causing either little analgesic effect in poor metabolisers or adverse side effects in ultra-rapid metabolisers. It is inappropriate to switch from Codeine to another weak opioid if pain is not well-controlled. Morphine should be used instead. Morphine has no ceiling dose while Codeine has a dose limit of 240 mg per day, which is equivalent to 24 mg of Morphine per day.

Other reported indications for Codeine include cough and diarrhoea.

WHAT ARE THE SIDE EFFECTS OF CODEINE?

The side-effects are similar to Morphine. It can cause more constipation than other weak opioids. Equivalent doses of Morphine may be less constipating. Laxatives should be prescribed prophylactically.

Note: Caution is needed in renal failure as the active metabolites can accumulate.

HOW TO START CODEINE?

- The starting dose may be 30 mg TDS, which can be increased up to 4-6 hourly. The maximum dose is 240 mg/day.
- The usual dose of Panadeine is 2 tabs TDS-QDS.

HOW TO DOSE CONVERT CODEINE TO MORPHINE?

Codeine is one-tenth the potency of Morphine. The ratio is 10:1.

Thus, if a patient is on 30 mg QDS of Codeine, the conversion from Codeine to Morphine is as follows:
- Step 1 : Total Codeine dose per day = 30 mg × 4 = 120 mg
- Step 2 : Converting Codeine to Morphine = 120 mg divided by 10 = 12 mg of Morphine daily
- Step 3 : This approximates to 2.5 mg Q4H of Morphine (~15 mg)

REFERENCES

1. Vallejo R, Barkin RL. Pharmacology of opioids in the management of chronic pain syndromes. *Pain Physician*. 2011;14(4):E343–360.
2. www.bpac.org.nz: WHO Analgesic Ladder: Which weak opioid to use at step two? 2008;18:20–23.

FENTANYL

Raphael Lee

WHAT IS FENTANYL?

Fentanyl is a highly lipophilic, synthetic strong opioid that acts predominantly on the μ-opioid receptor. It is already an active opioid in itself and is metabolised by the CYP3A4 enzyme predominantly in the liver and intestinal mucosa into inactive metabolites norfentanyl and hydroxyfentanyl, which are excreted through the kidneys.

It is more potent than Morphine.

WHAT ARE THE AVAILABLE FORMULATIONS?

- Transdermal Fentanyl Patch
  - Fentanyl 12 mcg/hr
  - Fentanyl 25 mcg/hr
  - Fentanyl 50 mcg/hr
- Sublingual tablets (Abstral®)
  - 100 mcg
  - 200 mcg
- Injectable Fentanyl
  - Fentanyl 100 mcg/2 ml
  - Fentanyl 500 mcg/10 ml

PRACTICAL TIPS

Transdermal Fentanyl takes about 8–12 hours to have its maximal effect after it has been applied, and has a similar residual effect of 8–12 hours after it is removed. It generally lasts for 72 hours.

Localisation influences fentanyl absorption because of differences in skin thickness and subcutaneous fat.

Recommended areas of application include the upper arms, thorax and upper back

Injectable Fentanyl can be given subcutaneously:

1. Onset: 15 minutes
2. Excreted: 30–60 minutes
   Therefore, breakthrough doses can be given hourly if necessary

Sublingual fentanyl (Abstral®) is indicated to manage breakthrough pain only in selected patients who are opioid tolerant ie consuming a morphine equivalent daily dose of 60mg for more than a week.

1. Onset: 10 mins
2. Initial treatment dose: 100 mcg 6H PRN
3. Titration: Increase sublingual fentanyl dose to 200 mcg 6H PRN if a dose of 100 mcg is insufficient for pain control
4. In the above scenario, no more than 2 doses of Abstral 100 mcg (spaced at least 30 mins apart) may be used to treat an episode of breakthrough pain

WHEN DO WE USE FENTANYL?

- Patients who cannot take orally (nausea and vomiting)
- Patients who have difficulty with compliance to oral Morphine
- Patients who develop side-effects or toxicity to Morphine and there is a need to opioid rotate
- Patients who have severe constipation with Morphine
- Patients with renal impairment (Cr Cl <30 ml/min) and liver impairment (ALT/AST > 3× upper limit of normal)

- Patients who are averse to Morphine but agreeable to use another strong opioid

WHAT ARE THE SIDE-EFFECTS OF FENTANYL?

As Fentanyl is a strong opioid, the side-effects are similar to that of Morphine — drowsiness and sedation. However, it causes less constipation as it does not act on gastrointestinal opioid receptors.

HOW TO START FENTANYL?

Due to its long duration of action, transdermal fentanyl is not suitable for patients with unstable pain. Titrate short acting opioids like immediate release morphine sulphate to achieve adequate pain control first before converting to a transdermal fentanyl patch.
- Transdermal Fentanyl Patch
  - Start Fentanyl 6 mcg/hr q72H (use half of a 12 mcg/hr Fentanyl patch)
- Fentanyl Infusion
  - Start at S/C Fentanyl 10 mcg/hr (Fentanyl 0.2 ml/hr)

HOW TO DOSE CONVERT FENTANYL TO MORPHINE?

- Fentanyl is more potent than Morphine. The equipotent ratio is 1:100
- Converting Morphine to Fentanyl
  Thus, if a patient is on Morphine 5 mg 4H:
  - Step 1 : Total Daily Morphine Requirement (24 hours) 5 mg × 6 = 30 mg
  - Step 2 : Converting Morphine from mg to mcg = 30 × 1,000 = 30,000 mcg
  - Step 3 : Converting Morphine to per hour = 30,000/24 = 1,250 mcg/hr
  - Step 4 : Converting Morphine to Fentanyl using equipotent ratio of 1:100 = 1,250/100 = 12.5 mcg/hr
- Start the patient on Fentanyl Patch 12 mcg/hr q72H

A Much Easier Way to Remember the Conversion Ratios Is to Use the Conversion Factor 2.4

Morphine to Fentanyl

- Morphine 5 mg 4 hourly = Total Daily Morphine $5 \times 6 = 30$ mg
- Fentanyl Requirement: $30/2.4 = 12.5$ mcg/hr

Fentanyl to Morphine

Similarly, for patients on Fentanyl 25 mcg/hr transdermal patch who need to convert to Oral Morphine:

- Fentanyl $25 \times 2.4 = 60$ mg per day of oral Morphine
- Order Morphine 10 mg q4H

HOW TO ORDER BREAKTHROUGH FENTANYL?

Whilst on a Fentanyl basal infusion, the breakthrough dose is 1/10th of the total Fentanyl dose (i.e. over 24 hours).

E.g. If basal dose of Fentanyl is 10 mcg/hr: Breakthrough (BT) dose is: $10 \times 24 = 240/10 = 24$ mcg. We order Fentanyl BT 25 mcg prn up to hourly.

REFERENCES

1. Cleary JF. The pharmacological management of cancer pain. *J Palliat Med.* 2007;10(6):1369–1374.
2. Rauck RL, Tark M, Reyes E, Hayes TG, Bartkowiak AJ, Hassman D, Nalamachu S, Derrick R, Howell J. Efficacy and long-term tolerability of sublingual fentanyl orally disintegrating tablet in the treatment of breakthrough cancer pain. *Curr Med Res Opin.* 2009 Dec;25(12):2877–2885.
3. Kuip EJ, Zandvliet ML, Koolen SL, Mathijssen RH, van der Rijt CC. A review of factors explaining variability in fentanyl pharmacokinetics; focus on implications for cancer patients. *Br J Clin Pharmacol.* 2017;83(2):294–313.

KETAMINE

Allyn Hum and Mahrley Tanagon Provido

WHAT IS KETAMINE?

Ketamine, at sub-anesthetic doses is a potent analgesic. It acts on N-methyl D-aspartate (NMDA) receptors which play an important role in mitigating tolerance to opioids, management of neuropathic pain and central sensitisation.

WHAT ARE THE AVAILABLE FORMULATIONS?

Ketamine is available in 500mg/10mL or 100mg/2mL formulations.

WHEN DO WE USE KETAMINE?

As a potent NMDA receptor antagonist, ketamine is involved in the desensitization of the wind-up phenomenon responsible for most neuropathic pain syndromes. It is best selected for use in patients demonstrating central sensitization. Ketamine has also been shown to be useful in treating major depression.

WHAT ARE THE ROUTES OF ADMINISTRATION?

Ketamine is usually administered orally or parenterally.

WHAT ARE THE SIDE-EFFECTS?

- Tachycardia, hypertension
- Hallucinations, vivid dreams, floating sensations, visual-spatial phenomena (psychomimetic side effects)
- Delirium, dizziness, diplopia, nystagmus, altered hearing
- Nausea, vomiting, anorexia, hypersalivation
- Urinary tract symptoms (frequency, urgency, urge incontinence, dysuria, hematuria)

WHAT ARE THE RELATIVE CONTRAINDICATIONS?

- Known hydrocephalus or raised intracranial pressure
- Recent history of epilepsy
- Severe systemic hypertension
- Severe psychiatric disorders

WHAT ARE THE DRUGS THAT MAY INTERACT?

Plasma concentrations of ketamine may be increased by diazepam. Ketamine may also affect metabolism of warfarin, phenytoin, theophylline (tachycardia and seizures) and levothyroxine (hypertension and tachycardia).

HOW TO START KETAMINE?

Subcutaneous route	"Burst" infusion	Oral formulation
1. Syringe out 75 mg of ketamine (1.5 mls) + 5 mg Haloperidol * (1 ml) and dilute with normal saline up to 24 mls and run at 1 mls per hour over 24 hours. 2. Reduce concurrent opioid dose by 30%.[†]	1. Start SC Ketamine infusion at 100 mg over 24 hours. 2. Increase to 300 mg after 24 hours if pain is suboptimal.	1. Starting dose of 10–25 mg TDS-QDS. 2. Increase by 10–25 mg up to 100 mg QDS (max. dose: 200 mg QDS).

(Continued)

Subcutaneous route	"Burst" infusion	Oral formulation
3. For patients with persistent pain after 24 hours, escalate ketamine dose by increments of 100 mg daily. 4. Continue infusion at the lowest effective dose needed to achieve analgesia. 5. After 5 days, convert to oral ketamine using a 1:1 ratio.	3. Further increase to 500 mg over 24 hours if it is still ineffective. 4. Stop three days after the last increment.	3. When converting from Parenteral Ketamine to Oral Ketamine, use a ratio of 1:1.[‡]

*Use of benzodiazepines, alpha-2 agonists, antidepressants, antihistamines, or anticholinergics prior to the initiation of ketamine as prophylaxis for psychomimetic side effects (grade C recommendation).

[†]Reduction of opioid consumption is explained by the effect of ketamine on pain-induced central sensitization. An alternative reason for this is the ability of NMDA receptor antagonists to inhibit acute tolerance to the analgesic effect of opioids.

[‡]Oral consumption of Ketamine results in smaller peak levels, which may result in less pronounced side-effects than when used parenterally. There are varying reports as to the equipotency between oral and subcutaneous Ketamine. The median range is 1:1.

REFERENCES

1. Provido-Aljibe MT, Yee CM, Carin Low ZJ, Hum A. The impact of a standardised ketamine step protocol for cancer neuropathic pain. *Prog Palliat Care*. 29(3):May 2021;doi:10.1080/09699260.2021.1922146.
2. Chapman EJ, Edwards Z, Boland JW, Maddocks M, Fettes L, Malia C, *et al.* Practice review: Evidence-based and effective management of pain in patients with advanced cancer. *Palliat Med*. 2020;34(4):444–453.

3. Bredlau AL, Thakur R, Korones DN, Dworkin RH. Ketamine for pain in adults and children with cancer: A systematic review and synthesis of the literature. *Pain Med*. 2013;14(10):15051

4. Prommer EE. Ketamine: Making sense of multiple routes and protocols. *J Pain Symptom Manage*. 2012;43(2):331–332.

5. Hardy J, Quinn S, Fazekas B, Plummer J, Eckermann S, Agar M, *et al*. Randomized, double-blind, placebo-controlled study to assess the efficacy and toxicity of subcutaneous ketamine in the management of cancer pain. *J Clin Oncol*. 2012;30(29):3611–3617.

6. Benítez-Rosario MA, Salinas-Martín A, González-Guillermo T, Feria M. A strategy for conversion from subcutaneous to oral ketamine in cancer pain patients: Effect of a 1:1 ratio. *J Pain Symptom Manage*. 2011;41(6): 1098–1105

7. Jackson K, Ashby M, Martin P, Pisasale M, Brumley D, Hayes B. "Burst" Ketamine for refractory cancer pain: An open-label audit of 39 patients. *J Pain Symptom Manage*. 2001;22(4):834–842.

8. Kissin I, Bright CA, Bradley EL. The effect of ketamine on opioid-induced acute tolerance: Can it explain reduction of opioid consumption with ketamine-opioid analgesic combinations? *Anesth Analg*. 2000;91(6): 1483–1488.

METHADONE

Allyn Hum and Mahrley Tanagon Provido

WHAT IS METHADONE?

Methadone as a synthetic μ-opioid agonist plays an integral part in the management of cancer pain for the following reasons:

- Multiple receptor affinities (μ, ∂ & NMDA) resulting in additive analgesic control and limiting opioid tolerance
- Good oral bioavailability (~40–99%)
- Absence of active metabolites that produce neurotoxicity
- Clearance independent of renal function
- Cost effectiveness

LIMITATION OF USE

- Long and unpredictable half-life
- Drug interactions as its metabolism is via the cytochrome P450 group of enzymes

WHAT ARE THE AVAILABLE FORMULATIONS?

- Methadone is available in 5mg scored tablets. Unlike other sustained-released opioids, it can be 'cut' into half which is equivalent to 2.5 mg
- A ratio of 1:2 is used to convert parental Methadone which can be given intravenously or subcutaneously, to tablets via oral route

- Rectal Methadone (in a liquid form and given as an enema) has also been used

WHEN DO WE USE METHADONE?

- As a 3rd or 4th line opioid when pain continues to be sub-optimally controlled, or when side-effects of the preceding opioid outweigh benefits
- When pain is not well-controlled by high doses of conventional opioids
- For opioid rotation due to side-effects of other opioids
- For predominantly neuropathic pain
- As an adjuvant/co-analgesic to low dose opioids in the management of complex pain

HOW TO CONVERT TO METHADONE?

Unlike most opioids, the equianalgesic conversion of Methadone is relatively unstable and unpredictable. Equianalgesic ratios between Morphine and Methadone are based on the Morphine equivalent daily dose (MEDD) i.e. the dose ratio of Methadone to Morphine is inversely proportional to the daily Morphine dose administered.

A fixed equianalgesic ratio of 10:1 may be adequate for patients at low-to-moderate MEDD <400 mg/day

Morphine Equivalent Daily Dose (MEDD)	Morphine : Methadone
≤ 1000 mg/day	10 : 1
>1000 mg/day	30 : 1

OPIOID ROTATION TO METHADONE

1. **Stop and Go Method**
   - For patients with an opioid requirement of Morphine Equivalent Daily Dose (MEDD) 100mg or less
   - To STOP the existing opioid completely and GO with the target dose of Methadone immediately in 2–3 divided doses per day

Thus, for a patient with an MEDD of 70mg, the Morphine to Methadone conversion is as follows:

Step 1. 70mg divided by 10 (using equianalgesic ratio of 10:1) = 7 mg of Methadone

Step 2. Decrease by 30% for incomplete cross tolerance = 5 mg/day of Methadone (target dose) given in 2 divided doses

2. **3-Day Method**
   - For patients with an opioid requirement of MEDD more than 100 mg
   - Allows for adjustment to the variable pharmacokinetics and unique pharmacodynamics of methadone

Opioid	Day 1	Day 2	Day 3	Day 4
Morphine (Example)	Reduce by ⅓	Reduce by a further ⅓	Cease Morphine	—
Methadone	Start at ⅓ of target dose	Increase to ⅔ of target dose	Full dose	Full dose
Breakthrough Opioid	⅙–¹⁄₁₀ th of the original opioid	⅙–¹⁄₁₀ th of the original opioid	⅙–¹⁄₁₀ th of the original opioid	⅙–¹⁄₁₀ th of the original opioid

Thus, for a patient with MEDD of 200mg, the Morphine to Methadone conversion is as follows:

Step 1. 200 mg divided by 10 (using equianalgesic ratio of 10:1) = 20 mg/day of Methadone

Step 2. Decrease by 30% for incomplete cross tolerance = 15 mg/day of Methadone (target dose) given in 3 divided doses

Opioid	Day 1	Day 2	Day 3	Day 4
Morphine	135 mg/ day (⅓ reduction)	66 mg/day (further ⅓ reduction)	Cease Morphine	—
Methadone	5 mg/day (⅓ target dose)	10 mg/day (⅔ target dose)	15 mg/day (target dose)	**15 mg/day** (given in 3 divided doses)

WHAT ARE THE SIDE-EFFECTS?

The side-effects of Methadone are similar to that of opioids. However, Methadone has a long half-life and has many drug interactions that may lead to toxicity.

WHAT ARE THE DRUGS THAT MAY INTERACT WITH METHADONE?

These are the medications that may interact with Methadone when co-administered.

Decrease Methadone Levels	Increase Methadone Levels
Antibiotics • Rifampicin	Cimetidine Ciprofloxacin
Anticonvulsants • Phenytoin • Phenobarbitone • Carbamazepine	Fluconazole Fluoxetine Ketoconazole Macrolides
Psychotropics • Risperidone	Nifedipine Sertraline
Antiretrovirals • Ritonavir • Nevirapine	TCAs Zidovudine

PRACTICAL TIP

1. Rotating to Methadone should only be done after consulting a senior palliative care physician versed in its use.

REFERENCES

1. Tan C, Wong CF, Yee CM, Hum A. Methadone rotation for cancer pain: An observational study, *BMJ Support Palliat Care*. 2020:01–4.
2. Reddy A, Yennurajalingam S *et al*. Dual opioid therapy using methadone as a co-analgesic. *Expert Opin Drug Saf*. 2015 Jan;14(1):181–182.
3. Leppert W. The role of methadone in cancer pain treatment — A review. *Int J Clin Pract*. 2009;63:1095–1109.
4. Ripamonti C, Bianchi M. The use of Methadone for cancer pain. *Haematol Oncol Clin North Am*. 2002;16:543–555.
5. Weschules DJ, Bain KT. A systematic review of opioid conversion ratios used with Methadone for the treatment of pain. *Pain Med*. 2008;9(5):595–612.
6. Bruera E, Palmer JL *et al*. Methadone versus Morphine as a first-line strong opioid for cancer pain: A randomised, double-blind study. *J Clin Oncol*. 2004;22(1):185–192.

MORPHINE

Mervyn Koh and Lee Hwei Khien

WHAT IS MORPHINE?

Morphine is the commonest strong opioid used in managing cancer pain. It is the prototype opioid agonist that acts mainly on μ-opioid receptors but it also has effects on ∂ and k-opioid receptors. Morphine sulphate undergoes hepatic glucuronidation to form primarily Morphine-6-glucuronide (M6G) (10–15%) and Morphine-3-glucuronide (M3G) (55–80%).

M6G is the active analgesic component while M3G does not have any analgesic properties. M3G may be responsible for the undesirable neuroexcitatory side-effects like hyperalgesia, allodynia and myoclonus. Both are excreted by the kidneys.

WHAT ARE THE AVAILABLE MORPHINE FORMULATIONS IN SINGAPORE?

Oral	• Liquid: Morphine (also known as mist morphine • 1 mg/mL (e.g. Statex®, RAmorph®)* • 2 mg/mL (e.g. Oramorph®)**

(Continued)

235

(*Continued*)

	• Tablet: Morphine Sulphate Sustained-Release Tablets (MST): MST Continus® 10mg/30mg Tablets[†] [†]*Do not cut/crush sustained-release tablets*
Injectable	Each 1 ml-Ampoule contains 10 mg of Morphine Sulphate, which can be given subcutaneously or intravenously

*Safety considerations:
- There are two concentrations (1 mg/mL and 2 mg/mL) of Mist morphine registered in Singapore in Y2020.
- When performing a medication review, always check the concentration the patient is taking.

Morphine	Mist Morphine	MST Continus®	Morphine (SC)	Morphine (IV)
Onset of Action	30 min	Not available	15 min	5 min
Maximal Effect	60 min	1–5 hr	50–90 min	10–20 min
Duration of Action	3–6 hr	8–12 hr	4–6 hr	4–6 hr

WHEN DO WE USE MORPHINE?

It is used for the treatment of moderate to severe cancer pain, as well as for dyspnea.

WHAT ARE THE COMMON SIDE-EFFECTS OF MORPHINE?

The common side-effects include constipation, nausea, vomiting, sedation and confusion. ALL patients on Morphine need to be on laxatives (see the section on Constipation). The other side-effects can be minimised by starting Morphine at lower doses. Even if they do occur, these effects are usually transient and resolve within a few days.

Morphine 'toxicity' which manifests as myoclonic jerks, 'pinpoint pupils' and respiratory depression (Respiratory Rate <8/ min) is uncommon when used in correct doses and titrated upwards carefully.

HOW TO START ORAL MORPHINE?

- Starting dose of Mist Morphine is usually 2.5–5 mg 4–6 hourly
- In the elderly where we anticipate delayed hepatic metabolism and renal excretion, we can reduce the dose further to 2.5 mg 8 hourly

HOW TO START PARENTERAL MORPHINE?

Morphine should only be given parenterally (SC or IV) when symptoms (pain or dyspnea) are severe and/or need to be controlled rapidly (e.g. in an imminently dying patient).

- Give SC/IV Morphine 2.5 mg 'stat' followed by a basal infusion
- SC/IV Morphine 0.2–1 mg/hr (Dilute 10 mg of Morphine in Normal Saline to make up to 10 ml = 1 mg/ml)

HOW TO ORDER BREAKTHROUGH MORPHINE?

Patients on regular Morphine should have Morphine on standby for breakthrough pain. This is usually 1/6th of the total daily Morphine dose.
  Thus, for a patient who is on Mist Morphine 5 mg 4 hourly:
— Step 1: Calculate the total Oral Morphine required per day
   — 5 mg × 6 = 30 mg of Mist Morphine per day
— Step 2: Calculate Breakthrough Dose (1/6th of total daily Morphine dose)
   — 30 mg/6 = 5 mg of Morphine

HOW TO DECIDE ON THE FREQUENCY OF BREAKTHROUGH DOSES?

- Usually, the dosing frequency is four or six hourly. Generally, the interval in between breakthrough doses would be four hours less than the regular dose

- Thus, for a patient who is on Mist Morphine 5 mg 4 hourly: Breakthrough dose would be 5mg PRN (up to 4 hourly) only when necessary

MUST WE ADJUST THE DOSE OF MORPHINE IN HEPATIC AND RENAL IMPAIRMENT?

- In renal (CrCl < 30 mL/min) or hepatic impairment (AST/ALT >3 times upper limit of normal), the dose should be reduced by half. Increasing the dosing interval can be attempted as drug elimination is reduced. Opioid rotation to Fentanyl should also be considered
- If CrCl < 10 ml/min, rotate to Fentanyl

DOSE CONVERSION FROM ORAL TO PARENTERAL MORPHINE

- The conversion ratio from Oral to Parenteral Morphine is 3:1
- Thus, if a patient is on Mist Morphine 5 mg 4 hourly and develops vomiting or can no longer consume orally and requires conversion to Parenteral Morphine:
  - Step 1 : Calculate the total Oral Morphine required per day
    - 5 mg × 6 = 30 mg of Mist Morphine per day
  - Step 2 : Convert Oral to Parenteral Morphine (3:1)
    - 30 of Oral Morphine: 10 mg of Parenteral Morphine per day
  - Step 3 : Convert to Morphine (SC/IV) Infusion
    - 10 mg/24hr = 0.4 mg of Morphine per hour

REFERENCES

1. Cleary JF. The pharmacological   management of cancer pain. *J Palliat Med.* 2007;10(6):1369–1394.
2. Wilcock A., *et al. Palliative Care Formulary.* 7th Ed.
3. MST Continus® Product Insert. Bard Pharmaceuticals Limited.

OXYCODONE

Mervyn Koh and Lee Hwei Khien

WHAT IS OXYCODONE?

Oxycodone is a synthetic opioid that interacts with both μ and κ receptors but is similar to Morphine in many aspects.

Oxycodone is metabolised in the liver by CYP3A4 to noroxycodone and by CYP2D6 to oxymorphone respectively, both of which possess analgesic activity. Oxycodone itself exerts its analgesic effects with negligible contribution from its active metabolites. They are subsequently excreted by the kidneys. Oxycodone, like Morphine, needs to be used with caution in hepatic and renal impairment.

Oxycodone is 1.5 to 2 times more potent than oral Morphine and it remains a paradox that Oxycodone has high analgesic potency despite a relatively low affinity for μ receptors compared to Morphine.

Oxycodone has similar side-effects as Morphine.

WHAT ARE THE AVAILABLE FORMULATIONS IN SINGAPORE?

- It comes in three different oral formulations:
  - Immediate release (Oxynorm®) 5 mg, 10 mg, 20 mg capsules and 1 mg/ml oral solution
  - Controlled-release (Oxycontin® Neo) 10 mg and 20 mg tablets (which actually contains 40% immediate-release and 60% controlled release Oxycodone, therefore leading to a biphasic drug release with an initial fast onset of action)

— Targin® Prolonged Release Tablets which contains oxycodone/naloxone in a fixed 2:1 ratio. Available strengths are 5 mg/2.5 mg, 10 mg/5 mg, 20 mg/10 mg, 40 mg/20 mg, 60 mg/30 mg, 80 mg/40 mg

Oxycodone	Immediate Release	Modified* Release
Onset	30–60 min	30–60 min
Peak	60–90 min	1.5–3 hr
Duration	3–6 hr	12 hr

*Modified release include both prolonged and extended release formulations.

- Parenteral Oxycodone (SC/IV) is half the dose of Oral Oxycodone e.g. Oxycodone 20 mg PO = Oxycodone 10 mg SC/IV

WHEN DO WE USE OXYCODONE-CONTAINING PRODUCTS?

- Patients who are averse to Morphine but are otherwise agreeable to the use of strong opioids
- Patients who have side-effects to Morphine and require opioid rotation
- Like Morphine, Oxycodone should be used with caution in patients with hepatic and renal impairment

WHEN DO WE USE TARGIN®?

- Targin® can be considered for patients who experience persistent opioid-induced constipation despite laxative use
- The naloxone content in Targin® acts locally at the opioid receptors in the gastrointestinal tract without affecting the bioavailability and analgesic effect of oxycodone
- Constipation can still occur with Targin® but at a lower incidence rate. Therefore, laxatives should still be prescribed

WHAT ARE THE SIDE-EFFECTS OF OXYCODONE-CONTAINING PRODUCTS?

The side-effects of Oxycodone are similar to that of Morphine.

HOW TO START OXYCODONE?

Oxycodone should not be started as first-line agents in opioid naïve patients. However, if really necessary, start immediate-release Oxynorm 5 mg q8H–q6H.

Once optimal analgesic dose has been established, consideration can be made to convert to a controlled-release formulation to reduce the need for multiple dosing.

HOW TO CONVERT THE DOSE OF MORPHINE TO OXYCODONE?

- If a patient is on Morphine Sulphate slow release 100 mg q12H, then the conversion from Morphine to Oxycodone is as follows:
  - Step 1 : Total daily Oral Morphine requirement (24 hours) 100 mg × 2 = 200 mg
  - Step 2 : Converting Morphine to Oxycodone (2:1) = 200 mg : 100 mg of Oxycodone. Reduce further by 30% to account for incomplete cross tolerance. Eventual dose of Oxycodone: 70 mg/day
  - Step 3 : Hence prescribe Oxycodone sustained released (Oxycontin Neo®) 40 mg OM, 30 mg ON, 12 hours apart

HOW TO ORDER BREAKTHROUGH OXYCODONE?

- If a patient needs Oxycodone 100 mg over 24 hours, then ordering breakthrough Oxycodone is as follows:
  - Step 1 : Calculate one-sixth of total daily dose for each breakthrough dose, i.e. 16.6 mg of Oxycodone
  - Step 2 : Hence prescribe Oxycodone immediate release (Oxynorm) 15 mg prn, max. 4 hourly (Use Oxynorm 5 mg × 3)

PRACTICAL TIPS

1. Never crush sustained release Oxycodone (Oxycontin) tablets. The dose of Oxycodone meant to be released over a period of 12 hours will peak within 1 hour.

REFERENCES

1. Cleary JF. The pharmacological management of cancer pain. *J Palliat Med.* 2007;10(6):1369–1394.
2. Targin Prolonged Release Tablet Product Insert. Mundipharma Pharmaceuticals Pte Ltd.
3. Ahmedzai SH, *et al.* Long-term safety and efficacy of oxycodone/naloxone prolonged-release tablets in patients with moderate-to-severe chronic cancer pain. *Support Care Cancer.* 2015;23:823–830.

TRAMADOL

Chia Siew Chin

WHAT IS TRAMADOL?

Tramadol is a centrally-acting analgesic with opioid and non-opioid properties. It acts on the μ-opioid receptor after conversion to the active metabolite, O-desmethyltramadol. It also stimulates neuronal serotonin release and inhibits the pre-synaptic re-uptake of serotonin and noradrenaline.

Further metabolism produces inactive metabolites that are excreted via the kidneys.

WHAT ARE THE AVAILABLE FORMULATIONS?

- Tramadol can come in the form of:
  - Oral Tramadol, which comes in two oral forms — a 50 mg tablet which can be halved, and a 50 mg capsule
  - Injectable Tramadol 50 mg/ml given intravenously or intramuscularly
  - A combination with Paracetamol, i.e. Ultracet: Tramadol 37.5 mg and Paracetamol 325 mg
- Onset of action: 30 min–1 hour
- Duration of action: 4–8 hours

WHEN DO WE USE TRAMADOL?

It is used for pain of moderate intensity.

In placebo-controlled trials (done in diabetic neuropathy, post-herpetic neuralgia and polyneuropathy), it improves neuropathic pain. However, in an RCT of cancer/non-cancer patients with or without neuropathic pain, it is no different from Morphine.

WHAT ARE THE SIDE-EFFECTS OF TRAMADOL?

It has similar side-effects as other opioids. Compared to Morphine, it causes less constipation and respiratory depression. However, it causes more giddiness, vomiting and anorexia than Codeine or Morphine.

It is contraindicated in patients on Monoamine Oxidase Inhibitors (MAOIs), in patients with CrCl <10 mL/min, and in uncontrolled epilepsy.

WHAT DRUG INTERACTIONS ARE POSSIBLE?

Care should be taken when there is concurrent administration of medication which lowers the seizure threshold, e.g. TCAs, SSRIs and antipsychotics.

Caution should also be exercised when there is concurrent administration of medications which interfere with pre-synaptic serotonin reuptake, e.g. Selective Serotonin Reuptake Inhibitors (SSRIs). This may lead to Serotonin Syndrome (confusion, autonomic hyperactivity such as tachycardia, blood pressure changes, fever and neuromuscular changes such as tremor and rigidity).

HOW TO START TRAMADOL?

- The starting dose of Oral Tramadol is 50 mg TDS-QDS, although we can start at 25 mg TDS for frail, elderly patients
- The maximum dose is 400 mg/day, although for the elderly (>75 years old), it should not exceed 300 mg/day

- In renal (CrCl <30 mL/min) or hepatic impairment, the dosing should be reduced to 50 mg 12 hourly, and the dose should not exceed 150 mg/day
- Tramadol injections can be given at 50–100 mg, 6 hourly

HOW TO CONVERT THE DOSE OF TRAMADOL TO MORPHINE?

Injectable Tramadol is one-tenth as potent as Oral Morphine. Studies have shown that oral Tramadol is one-fifth as potent as Oral Morphine, but some clinicians will regard the potency to be one-tenth (similar to injectable Tramadol). For frail and elderly patients, it may be safer to use the one-tenth conversion.

Thus, if a patient is on 50 mg TDS of Tramadol, the conversion from Tramadol to Morphine is as follows:

— Step 1 : 50 mg × 3 = 150 mg of Tramadol per day
— Step 2 : 150 mg of Tramadol is equivalent to 15 mg of Oral Morphine (10:1) or 30 mg of Oral Morphine (5:1)

REFERENCE

1. Vallejo R, Barkin RL. Pharmacology of opioids in the management of chronic pain syndromes. *Pain Physician*. 2011;14(4):E343–360.

LIGNOCAINE

Chia Siew Chin

WHAT IS LIGNOCAINE?

Lignocaine is an amide anaesthetic often used as analgesia, especially in neuropathic pain. At subanaesthetic doses, it blocks sodium channels, leading to decreased neuronal excitability and hence, less neuropathic pain and hyperalgesia without interfering with the normal function of sensory or motor neurons. It has also been shown to demonstrate anti-inflammatory properties, reduce central sensitization and decrease NMDA receptor-mediated post-synaptic depolarization.

WHAT ARE THE AVAILABLE FORMULATIONS?

Lignocaine may come in the form of:

- Parenteral Lignocaine given intravenously or subcutaneously as a bolus or infusion
- Topical Lignocaine 5% Patch for use in localized neuropathic pain, especially in allodynia or in gel form for use on the skin
- Oropharyngeal Lignocaine mouthwash or gargle for mucositis

In this chapter, we will concentrate on the use of Parenteral Lignocaine.

WHEN DO WE USE LIGNOCAINE?

Parenteral lignocaine can be used as an adjunct to opioids, similar to other neuropathic agents, and are useful:

- If the patients are unable to swallow oral neuropathic medications.
- As 'opioid-sparing' agents in patients at risk of developing opioid toxicity or in patients not responding to opioids
- In patients too ill to undergo invasive pain interventions
- As an alternative to the use of ketamine, which can precipitate delirium.

WHAT ARE THE SIDE EFFECTS OF LIGNOCAINE?

Lignocaine has a very narrow therapeutic index. The central nervous system (CNS) side effects may occur at a plasma level slightly above the therapeutic plasma level. Patients may experience CNS side effects before they experience any cardiovascular (CVS) side effects, as CVS side effects tend to occur at a much higher plasma level. If the patient experiences CNS side effects, discontinuing the lignocaine infusion in time may prevent the occurrence of CVS side effects.

CNS side effects include: tinnitus, perioral numbness, giddiness, delirium, drowsiness, seizures

CVS side effects include: cardiac arrhythmias, vascular tone changes (hypertension often precedes hypotension)

HOW TO START LIGNOCAINE?

A test dose of Lignocaine 100 mg (approximately 1–3 mg/kg) is commonly used to determine if the patient's pain is responsive to Lignocaine. This can be given subcutaneously as a slow bolus: 100 mg Lignocaine diluted with normal saline to 20 ml to run over 1 hour.

If deemed effective, a subcutaneous continuous infusion of 0.5 mg–2 mg/kg/hour may be run over 24 hours. A dose of 1200 mg/24 hours is often used as an initial starting dose, and the dose can be titrated to a maximum of 2 mg/kg/hour.

During the infusion, patients will be monitored for any changes in blood pressure, heart rate or CNS side effects.

It is postulated that the lignocaine dose–response curves for pain relief are characterized by a 'break point' in dosage, below which pain persists and above which pain is reduced. Conversely, the lignocaine dose remains stable over time if titrated to the dose that maintains adequate pain relief.

REFERENCES

1. Ferrini R, Paice JA. How to initiate and monitor infusional lidocaine for severe and/or neuropathic pain. *J Support Oncol.* 2004;2:90–94.
2. Chia SC, Hum A, Ong WY, Lee A. Parenteral Lignocaine in cancer neuropathic pain: A series of case reports. *Progress Palliat Care.* 2014;22(5);253–257.

SECTION 10: PRACTICAL ISSUES IN PALLIATIVE CARE

OPIOID CONVERSION CHART

Mervyn Koh and Christina Tan

Table 1: Opioid Conversion Chart (MILD OPIOIDS) Tan Tock Seng Palliative Medicine

Opioid	Starting Dose (mg)	Oral Morphine Equivalent	Frequency	Maximal Dose	Available Formulations
Panadeine (Paracetamol 500 mg/ Codeine 8 mg)	2 tabs	1.5 mg	6–8 hourly	2 tabs (6 hourly)	1 tab
Codeine*	30 mg	3 mg	6–8 hourly	60 mg (6 hourly)	30 mg
Tramadol*	50 mg	5–10 mg	6–8 hourly	100 mg (6 hourly)	50 mg

*Consider lower dose of codeine 15–30 mg and tramadol 25–50 mg in the elderly or in the presence of renal/hepatic impairment.

Table 2: Opioid Conversion Chart (STRONG OPIOIDS) Tan Tock Seng Palliative Medicine

Strong Opioid	Starting Dose (mg)	Oral Morphine Equivalent	Frequency	Maximal Dose	Available Formulations
Oxycodone*	5 mg	7.5–10 mg	4–6 hourly	No maximum	5 mg/10 mg CR/20 mg CR
Fentanyl Transdermal Patch[†]	12 mcg/hr	30 mg/24hr	q 72 hr	No maximum	12/25/50 mcg/hr
Fentanyl Sublingual Tablet (Abstral®)[‡]	100 mcg	—	2 hourly (max 4 doses/day)	800mcg up to 4 times a day	Not in TTSH formulary
Morphine Sulphate Mixture	2.5 mg	—	4–6 hourly	No maximum	1 mg/ml or 2 mg/ml
Morphine Sulphate Prolonged Release Tablets (MST Continus®)[†]	10 mg	—	12 hourly	No maximum	10 mg/ 30 mg
Morphine Sulphate injection (IV or S/C)	1 mg	3 mg	—	No maximum	10 mg/ml

Note:

* Oxycodone is available in the following formulations — Oxycodone Immediate-Release (Oxynorm) 5 mg capsules, or Oxycodone Controlled-Release (Oxycontin Neo®) 10 and 20 mg tablets, or in combination with prolonged-release naloxone (Targin® Prolonged Release 5mg/2.5mg tablets).

[†] Long-acting opioids including Fentanyl patch and Morphine SR tablets should not be started as first-line opioids in opioid-naïve patients.

[‡] Fentanyl Sublingual tablet is only indicated for treatment of breakthrough cancer pain in **opioid-tolerant** patients. Do NOT switch from other fentanyl containing products at a 1:1 ratio; a new dose titration with Abstral is required.

¶ Pethidine is NOT RECOMMENDED for use as an analgesic. It should not be used in the elderly or renal impaired patients as they have potent metabolites with unpredictably long half-lives which lower seizure threshold.

‖ Methadone usage is complicated. Please consult a palliative care or pain physician.

** Buprenorphine (Sovenor®) transdermal patch is available in TTSH but is rarely used in the palliative care setting as it is indicated only for treatment of chronic non-malignant pain.

CONTINUOUS SUBCUTANEOUS INFUSION DRUG CHART

Christina Tan

FOR COMMONLY PRESCRIBED DRUGS IN PALLIATIVE CARE

Drug	Indications	Availability	Dilution	Remarks
Buscopan (Hyoscine Butylbromide)	• Increased throat secretions • Anti-spasmodic	Injection: • 20 mg/ml	• Prescribed dose to be diluted in 0.9% saline to a total volume of 24 ml • To be infused over 24 hours at 1 ml/hr **Recommended Starting Dose:** To infuse Buscopan 40 mg over 24 hours, dilution will be: Buscopan 40 mg/2ml + 22 ml 0.9% Saline (Total volume after dilution = exactly 24 ml)	• Recommended maximum infusion dose is 120 mg/day
Fentanyl	• Dyspnea • Pain	Injection: • 100 mcg/ 2 ml • 500 mcg/ 10 ml	• Use 500 mcg/10ml vial for infusion • Use neat or undiluted • 50 mcg = 1 ml	• High alert medication • Drug of choice in hepatic and/or renal impairment • No ceiling to dose escalation

Recommended Starting Dose:
Fentanyl 10 mcg/hr

Converting routes of administration:
- To remove transdermal Fentanyl Patch when converting to parenteral infusion route
- If converting from parenteral to transdermal Fentanyl Patch, stop infusion 8 hours after applying patch due to delayed onset of effect from patch

---

Glycopyrrolate (Glycopyrronium)

- Increased throat secretions
- Anti-spasmodic

Injection:
- 0.6 mg/3 ml

- Prescribed dose to be diluted in 0.9% saline to a total volume of 24 ml
- To be infused over 24 hours at 1 ml/hr

Recommended Starting Dose:
To infuse Glycopyrrolate 1.2 mg over 24 hours, dilution

- Has less effect on heart rate compared to Buscopan
- Drug of choice in patients with tachycardia
- Recommended maximum dose is 2.4 mg/day

(Continued)

(Continued)

Drug	Indications	Availability	Dilution	Remarks
Haloperidol	• Nausea • Vomiting • Agitation • Restlessness	Injection: • 5 mg/ml	will be: Glycopyrrolate 1.2 mg/6 ml + 18 ml 0.9% Saline Total volume after dilution = exactly 24 ml • Prescribed dose to be diluted in 0.9% saline to a total volume of 24 ml • To be infused over 24 hours at 1 ml/hr **Recommended Starting** **Dose:** To infuse Haloperidol 5 mg over 24 hours, dilution will be: Haloperidol 5 mg/ml + 23 ml 0.9% Saline Total volume after dilution = exactly 24 ml	• Drug of choice for nausea and vomiting in complete intestinal obstruction • May not be very useful beyond 10 mg/day • Recommended maximum infusion dose is 20 mg/day • Haloperidol may precipitate at concentrations ≥ 1 mg/ml when diluted with 0.9% saline

| Ketamine | • Adjuvant for neuropathic pain through antagonism at the NMDA receptor

Note: NMDA stands for N-methyl-d-aspartate | Injection:
• 100 mg/ 2 ml (single-dose vial)
• 500 mg/ 10 ml (multi-dose vial) | • Prescribed dose to be given in combination with haloperidol or midazolam
• Mixture to be diluted with 0.9% saline to a total volume of 24 ml.
• To be infused over 24 hours at 1 ml/hr

Recommended Starting Dose:
Ketamine 75 mg/1.5 ml + Haloperidol 5 mg/ml + 21.5 ml 0.9% Saline
Total volume after dilution = exactly 24 ml
• Dose increase by 100 mg after 24 hrs if inadequate response | • High alert medication
• Recommended maximum infusion dose is 500 mg per day
• Use opioid analgesic for breakthrough
• Frequent monitoring of SC insertion site for redness or inflammation
• SC Dexamethasone 0.5–1 mg can be co-prescribed to reduce local inflammation of SC insertion site
• High risk for psychomimetic effects like euphoria, hallucinations, illusions and nightmares |

(Continued)

(Continued)

Drug	Indications	Availability	Dilution	Remarks
				• To start Haloperidol or Midazolam prophylactically for psychomimetic effects
Levetiracetam (also known as Keppra)	• Seizure	Injection: • 500 mg/5 ml	• Prescribed dose to be diluted in 0.9% saline to a total volume of 100 ml • To be infused over 12 hours **Recommended Starting Dose:** To infuse levetiracetam 1 g over 24 hours, dilute: Levetiracetam 500 mg/5 ml + 95 ml 0.9% Saline Total volume after dilution = exactly 100 ml Top-up infusion every 12 hourly.	• Recommended maximum dose is 3000 mg per day • Requires renal dose adjustment • Prepared as 12 H infusion to keep within max burette volume of 150ml

| Metoclopramide (Commonly known as Maxalon) | • Nausea
• Vomiting
• Prokinetic | Injection:
• 10 mg/2ml | • Prescribed dose to be diluted in 0.9% saline to a total volume of 24 ml
• To be infused over 24 hours at 1 ml/hr
Recommended Starting Dose:
To infuse Maxolon 30 mg over 24 hours, dilution will be:
Maxolon 30 mg/6ml + 18 ml 0.9% Saline
Total volume after dilution = exactly 24 ml | • Contraindicated in complete intestinal obstruction as increases risk of perforation
• Recommended maximum infusion dose is 1 mg/kg/day per day |
| Midazolam | • Anxiety
• Delirium
• Palliative sedation
• Seizures | Injection:
• 5 mg/5ml | • Use Midazolam 5 mg/5ml
• Use neat or undiluted
Recommended Starting Dose:
Midazolam 0.2–0.5 mg/hr (0.2–0.5 ml/hr) | • High alert medication
• Recommended maximum infusion dose is 100 mg per day
• May have to start at higher doses 0.5–1 mg/hr for palliative |

(Continued)

(Continued)

Drug	Indications	Availability	Dilution	Remarks
Morphine Sulfate	• Dyspnea • Pain	Injection • 10 mg/ml	• Dilute with 0.9% saline to concentration of 1 mg/ml Morphine Sulfate 10 mg/ml + 9 ml 0.9% Saline Total volume after dilution = exactly 10 ml (Conc: 1 mg/ml) **Recommended Starting Dose:** Morphine 0.2–0.5 mg/hr For patients on morphine infusion requiring breakthrough doses >2 mg: • DO NOT purge from syringe pump as volume exceeds 2 ml	sedation (consult a senior palliative physician) • High alert medication • Use with caution in hepatic and/or renal impairment due to risk of active metabolite accumulation • No ceiling to dose escalation

| Octreotide | Nausea
Vomiting
Anti-secretory effect | Injection:
• 100 mcg/ml | • Administer breakthrough dose separately using undiluted morphine
• Prescribed dose to be diluted in 0.9% saline to a total volume of 24 ml
• To be infused over 24 hours at 1 ml/hr

Recommended Starting Dose:
To infuse Octreotide 300 mcg over 24 hours, dilution will be:
Octreotide 300 mcg/3ml + 21 ml 0.9% Saline
Total volume after dilution = exactly 24 ml | • No breakthrough required
• Recommended maximum infusion dose is 900 mcg per day |
| Phenobarbital | • Seizures | Injection:
• 200mg/ml | • Prescribed dose to be diluted in 0.9% saline to a total volume of 48 ml
• To be infused over 24 hours at 2 ml/hr | • Larger volume of diluent to reduce site irritation as phenobarbital has high pH (10–11). |

(Continued)

(Continued)

Drug	Indications	Availability	Dilution	Remarks
			Recommended Starting Dose: To infuse Phenobarbital over 24 hours, dilution will be: Phenobarbital 400 mg/ 2 ml + 46 ml 0.9% Saline Total volume after dilution = exactly 48 ml	• Recommended max infusion dose is 2400 mg/day
Ranitidine	• Acid suppressant therapy • Reduce gastric secretion in malignant bowel obstruction	Injection: • 50mg/2ml	• Prescribed dose to be diluted in 0.9% saline to a total volume of 100 ml • To be infused over 24 hours	• Infuse using volumetric pump • Reduce to 100 mg/ 24 hours for CrCl < 50 ml/min • Monitor for confusion

Recommended Starting Dose:

To infuse Ranitidine 200mg over 24 hours, dilution will be:

Ranitidine 200 mg/8 ml + 92 ml 0.9% Saline

Total volume after dilution = exactly 100 ml

GENERAL INSTRUCTIONS

1. Infuse prescribed drugs via syringe pumps after dilution
2. Insert SC needle over the abdominal or thigh area if infused volume or breakthrough volume is more than 2 ml
3. Administer breakthrough via the 'purge' function of syringe pump for the following drugs:
   - Fentanyl
   - Morphine (if breakthrough volume ≤2 mg)
   - Midazolam
4. Administer breakthrough via bolus injection for the following drugs:
   - Buscopan (Hyoscine Butylbromide)
   - Glycopyrrolate (Glycopyrronium)
   - Haloperidol
   - Maxolon (Metoclopramide)
   - Morphine (if breakthrough volume >2 mg)
5. Bolus breakthrough volume should not exceed 2 ml
6. Insert additional SC port for bolus breakthroughs

DISCLAIMER NOTE

- This table refers to the use of sodium chloride 0.9% as diluent. Check with the pharmacist for compatibility if other diluents are used.
- Recommended maximum infusion doses may vary according to clinical situations. Always verify dosing with a senior palliative care clinical or pharmacist if in doubt.

REFERENCES

1. Dickman A, Schneider J. Varga J. *The Syringe Driver: Continuous Subcutaneous Infusions in Palliative Care*, 3rd ed. Oxford: Oxford University Press; 2011.
2. Twycross R, Wilcock A. *Palliative Care Formulary*, 3rd ed. Oxford: Radcliffe Publishing Ltd; 2007.
3. Back I. *Palliative Medicine Handbook*, 3rd ed.; 2001.
4. Storey P, Knight CF, Schonwetter RS. *Pocket Guide to Hospice/Palliative Medicine*. AAHPM; 2003.

HYPODERMOCLYSIS

Subcutaneous fluids may sometimes be used for maintaining hydration in patients who are:

- Unable to take adequate fluids orally
- Mildly to moderately dehydrated, and
- Lack of intravenous access

Preferred site: Abdomen/thigh area
Volume and rate: Maximum 1 L per SC site *(up to 1.5 L per SC site has been reported in literature)*

FLUIDS AND ADDITIVES

- Normal saline (0.9% NaCl)
- Dextrose 5%/Normal saline (0.9% NaCl)
- Dextrose 5% (limited experience locally, may have increased risk of site irritation/inflammation due to low pH of glucose)
- Dextrose 2.5%/0.45% NaCl

**Administration of potassium-containing drip via SC route has been reported in literature but we typically avoid its use due to concerns about local site reactions.

REFERENCES

1. Yap LK, Tan SH, Koo WH. Hypodermoclysis or subcutaneous infusion revisited. *Singapore Med J.* 2001;42(11):526–529.

2. UK Medicines Information Centre. Hypodermoclysis — Subcutaneous administration of fluids. UKMI Pharmacy News Volume 7; Number 4 December 2001. Available at: http://www.formulary.cht.nhs.uk/pdf,_doc_files_etc/Hospital_Policies/Bulletins/PharNews_Hypodermoclysis.pdf

DRUG COMPATIBILITY

Yee Choon Meng, Lee Hwei Khien, Christina Tan and Jade Wong

COMPATIBILITY OF DRUGS AND INFUSION OF MEDICATIONS

The mixing of drugs before administration generally constitutes "off label" prescribing and requires careful consideration. It is, however, inevitable at times when patients receiving palliative care require multiple medications for symptom relief, and are unable to take orally due to the following reasons:

- Inability to swallow (either dysphagia or too weak)
- Decreased level of consciousness
- Poor alimentary absorption
- Intractable vomiting
- Poor patient compliance

GENERAL PRINCIPLES

Care should be taken when mixing more than two drugs in a syringe and ensuring that the diluent used is compatible with the drugs. Although water for injection is used in many centres, it is hypotonic and may increase risk of site reactions. As such, sodium chloride 0.9% for injection is our preferred diluent of choice.

Syringe driver drug compatibility is often an empirical judgement, assessed based on a combination of visual appearance of the mixture and clinical assessment, when more robust chemical compatibility data is lacking. Lack of precipitate on mixing does not completely rule out incompatibility, hence clinical assessment must come hand-in-hand. For example, dexamethasone inactivates glycopyrrolate although no visual precipitate can be observed.

To minimize incompatibility, use a larger syringe to dilute the mixture to the maximum volume possible and keep the contents protected from light.

If more than three drugs are required in one syringe driver, re-assessment of treatment aims is required.

DRUG COMPATIBILITY CHART

Two-Drug Combinations

The following compatibility chart refers to the use of the two-drug combination diluted in sodium chloride 0.9% for 24 hours under ambient temperature, based on usual concentrations used in our practice.

When interpreting the compatibility chart, it is important to keep in mind that many factors affect compatibility, including the concentration of individual components, diluent used, order of mixing, temperature and storage duration after mixing.

For compatibility of three or more drug combinations or if the combination is not listed in the chart, consult a pharmacist or look up useful resources such as:

- Palliative Care Formulary Syringe Driver Survey Database (SDSD)
- Eastern Metropolitan Region Palliative Care Consortium Syringe Driver Drug Compatibilities
- Trissel's Clinical Pharmaceutics Database

	Buscopan (Hyoscine butyl-bromide)	Fentanyl	Glycopyrrolate	Ketamine	Haloperidol	Metoclopramide	Midazolam	Morphine sulphate	Octreotide	Ranitidine
Buscopan (Hyoscine butylbromide)										
Fentanyl	U									
Glycopyrrolate		U								
Ketamine	U	C²	U							
Haloperidol*	C¹	U	C²	C²						
Metoclopramide	C²,#	C²	C²,#	C²	C²					
Midazolam	U	C¹	C²	C²	C²	C²				
Morphine sulphate	U		C²	C¹	C²,@	C²	C¹			
Octreotide	U	U	U	U	C²	C²	U	C²		
Ranitidine	C²	U	U	U	U	C¹	I	C²	C²	

*Haloperidol is incompatible with NS at concentrations >1 mg/ml.

Legend:

C¹: Chemically compatible based on laboratory data

C²: Likely compatible based on either observational reports or physical/chemical compatibility data < 24hrs

U: Uncertain compatibility based on available data/no data

I: Incompatible

#: Prokinetic effect of metoclopramide may be inhibited by anticholinergics (buscopan, glycopyrrolate)

@: Dilute haloperidol with NS before mixing with morphine as the combination precipitates at high concentration

■: Agents from the same class should not be used together

REFERENCES

1. Dickman A, Schneider J, Varga J. *The Syringe Driver: Continuous Subcutaneous Infusions in Palliative Care*, 3rd ed. Oxford: Oxford University Press; 2011.
2. Back I. *Palliative Medicine Guidelines*. https://book.pallcare.info/index.php?tid=99&dg=9. Accessed on November 5, 2020.

TERMINAL DISCHARGE

Ang Ching Ching, Mervyn Koh and Wendy Ong

INTRODUCTION

An important element of achieving good end-of-life care is to honor patients' preferences. A high percentage of people indicate that home was their preferred place of death, with their family members giving it equal importance. Studies done in Singapore have also shown that most Singaporeans wish to die at home. As such, dying at home has been viewed as a vital component of a 'good death'.

'Terminal discharge' is the discharge of a dying patient with a short prognosis of hours to days. It is done to fulfil a patient's wish of dying at home. Ideally, it should be a planned process but more often than not, because of the unpredictability of the patient's condition, it may turn out to be a hurried one, causing tremendous stress to families and caregivers. Therefore, several considerations must be made prior to a terminal discharge.

CONSIDERATIONS BEFORE A TERMINAL DISCHARGE

Patient Factors

1. Desire to die at home
There is a need to consider the patient's expressed wish of dying at home, clarifying that the patient understands (if possible) that the discharge back home will imply a terminal event.

2.   Medical condition

Physicians will need to determine if there is any reversibility of the patient's current deterioration. It is important to prognosticate and identify this decline promptly so that well-timed conversations with regards to terminal discharge may be initiated with family members.

3.   Severity of symptoms and complications

Physicians will have to assess if the patient's symptoms can be managed at home. Difficult-to-manage symptoms and complications include seizures, massive bleeding and breathlessness from airway obstruction, potentially requiring palliative sedation. Refractory symptoms may increase the challenge of symptom management at home.

4.   Stability of the patient for transfer

In order to fulfil their loved ones' wishes, family members may insist on terminal discharge even when the patient is hypotensive or too unwell to be transferred. Hence, it is crucial that family members understand the possibility that the patient may die en-route home.

Family Members/Caregiver Factors

1.   Availability of caregivers

The care of a dying patient at home requires full-time caregivers who must be willing and ready to provide care. Family members may choose to take time off work or employ private nurses to assist with the nursing care of their loved ones at home.

2.   Ability to cope with care

Caring for a dying loved one or relative can cause significant stress on family members, both physically and emotionally. Nursing and medical care which is routine to healthcare professionals may be daunting for family members. Whilst grieving for the anticipated loss of their loved ones, family members must also be able to identify symptoms and administer medications. It is therefore necessary to provide caregiver training and assess if family members will be able to physically, and emotionally manage the patient's care at home.

3.   Understanding the intentions of a terminal discharge

Clear and honest communication is necessary to ensure that family members recognize the nature of the discharge as they may misunderstand the patient's discharge home as an improvement in their medical condition.

Involvement of Community Partners

1.   Referral to a home hospice care team

If the patient is known to a home hospice service provider, they must be contacted and informed about the plans for terminal discharge.

If the patient is not known to a home hospice service provider, a referral should be made if the terminal discharge takes place during weekdays and within office hours. Family members must be informed about the services provided by the home hospice care teams.

Providing an appropriate handover and proper documentation with detailed patient information is vital to ensure the continuity of care of the patient at home by the home hospice team.

2.   Private service providers

Terminal discharges during weekends and after office hours are discouraged as home hospice teams do not see new referrals during these periods. For patients who are not known to a home hospice team and are still keen for a terminal discharge during weekends and after office hours, family members will need to contact their private service providers (general practitioners or private home medical care services) to assist with medical support at home for the weekend.

PREPARATIONS FOR A TERMINAL DISCHARGE

Medications

- Consider the medications needed for symptom management, the doses required and if the routes of administration are appropriate
- Consider starting an infusion if the patient is symptomatic and no longer able to consume medications orally
- Ensure an adequate supply of medications (at least 3 days)

Equipment/Logistics

- Assist in the arrangement of an oxygen concentrator and/or other equipment rental if necessary
- Arrange for an ambulance, informing the ambulance officers regarding the nature of discharge

Caregiver Training

Provide education and training to family members and caregivers for the following:

- Administration of subcutaneous injections
- Nursing care, including oral hygiene, skin care, turning, maintenance of nasogastric tubes, indwelling catheters and wound dressing where necessary
- Signs of dying
- What to do when a loved one passes away at home

Documents

Provide the following documents:

- Discharge summary for the home hospice care team
- Memo to the general practitioner with the likely cause of death of the patient
- Memo to the ambulance officer stating the nature of discharge
- A list of community resources including private nursing agencies, general practitioners, vendors for family members to get medical equipment if necessary

REFERENCES

1. Schou-Andersen M, Ullersted M, Jensen BA, Neergaard MA, Factors associated with preference for dying at home among terminally ill patients with cancer. *J Caring Sci*. 2016;30:466–476.

2. Lin H-Y, Kang S-C, Chen Y-C, Chang Y-C, Wang W-S, Lo S-S, Place of death for hospice-cared terminal patients with cancer: A nationwide retrospective study in Taiwan. *J Chin Med Assoc.* 2017;80:227–232.

3. Gomes B, Calanzani N, Gysels M, Hall S, Higginson IJ. Heterogeneity and changes in preferences for dying at home: A systematic review. *BMC Palliat Care.* 2013;12 Article No. 7, https://doi.org/10.1186/1472-684X-12-7

4. Yao C-A, Hu W-Y, Lai Y-F, Cheng S-Y, Chen C-Y, Chiu T-Y. Does dying at home influence the good death of terminal cancer patients? *J Pain Symptom Manage.* 2007;34(5):497–504.

5. Lien Foundation (2014). Death Attitudes Survey.

6. Tan WS, Bajpai R, Ho AHY, Low CK, Car J. Retrospective cohort analysis of real-life decisions about end-of-life care preferences in a Southeast Asian country. *BMJ Open.* 2019; 9(2):e024662, https://doi.org/10.1136/bmjopen-2018-024662.

7. Merlene H, Booth Z. Discharge planning in end-of-life care. *Br J Nurs.* 2020;29(4):202–203.

8. Arias M, Garcia-Vivar C. The transition of palliative care from the hospital to the home: A narrative review of experiences of patients and family caretakers. *Invest Educ Enferm.* 2015;33(3):482–491.

9. Nyatanga B. Dying at home: Reconciling with patient and family wishes. *Br J Commun Nurs.* 2015;20(8):410.

OPIOID TOXICITY

Mervyn Koh and Allyn Hum

INTRODUCTION

The use of opioids for cancer and non-cancer pain or for other symptoms is well-established in palliative care.

In general, we should follow the principles of starting low, and going slow for opioid-naïve patients. However, in certain instances, either due to patient or medication related factors, patients may develop opioid toxicity.

SYMPTOMS

Patients can become delirious (either increasingly drowsy or excessively agitated) initially before developing myoclonic jerks, pinpoint pupils, and finally, respiratory depression (respiratory rate <8/min).

CAUSES

There could be several reasons leading to opioid toxicity, which may include:

1. Patient factors:
   Those who are at risk of:
   - Respiratory failure, especially those with Chronic Type 2 Respiratory Failure (Chronic Obstructive Lung Disease, neuromuscular disorders)

- Renal or liver impairment (Dehydration, especially in the elderly may worsen renal function and lead to toxicity)
- Infections

2. Medication factors:
   - Overly rapid escalation of opioids
   - Opioid rotation without factoring in incomplete cross tolerance (especially with Methadone due to its unpredictable half-life)

MANAGEMENT

If patients exhibit signs of toxicity, such as being overly-sedated, are delirious or develop myoclonic jerks, exclude modifiable causes such as an infection and discontinue other sedating drugs first.

If these measures do not resolve opioid toxicity, consider the following:

1. Reduce the opioid dose by 50% or consider opioid rotation
2. Have breakthrough (PRN) doses available
3. Re-hydrate the patient judiciously (1–2 litres of fluids)

INDICATIONS FOR NALOXONE

Naloxone, a competitive opioid antagonist, should only be used if there are life-threatening situations such as respiratory depression. Its half-life is between 30–60 minutes.

Indications for Naloxone:

- Respiratory Rate: <8/min
- Respiratory Rate: 8–12/min but unarousable (possible airway compromise)

Starting Dose: (Naloxone 0.4 mg/ml)

1. Dilute Naloxone in 10 ml Saline (0.04 mg/ml)
2. Administer IV 0.04–0.4 mg (depending on the opioid volume the patient was on, then observe for 2–5 minutes)

3. Escalate to the following doses if not better
   - IV 0.4 mg (then observe for another 2–5 minutes)
   - IV 2 mg
   - IV 4 mg

If not better after 10 mg of Naloxone, the cause of drowsiness is unlikely due to opioid toxicity.

MAINTENANCE INFUSION

An infusion of Naloxone (2/3 of the effective dose) may be necessary if there is an initial response to Naloxone but the patient subsequently becomes drowsy or develops respiratory compromise again.

E.g. If effective dose of Naloxone was 0.4 mg, then Naloxone Infusion should be 0.2–0.3 mg/hr.

PRACTICAL TIPS

1. When using opioids in patients at risk of toxicity, it may be more prudent to start at lower doses and use short-acting instead of long-acting formulations.
2. There is rarely a need in clinical practice to use Naloxone. Hydration and the reduction of the opioid dosage will usually suffice.
3. In case of emergency and a lack of venous access, Naloxone can also be given via IM or SC routes (0.4 mg).
4. Use of Intranasal and Nebulised Naloxone 0.8–2 mg has been described.

REFERENCES

1. Boyer E. Management of opioid analgesic overdose. *New Engl J Med.* 2012;367(2):146–155.
2. Hank G, Cherny NI, Fallon M. Opioid analgesic therapy. *Oxford Textbook of Palliative Medicine*, 3rd ed. Oxford University Press; 2003, p. 335.
3. Clark SF, Dargan PI, Jones AL. Naloxone in opioid poisoning: Walking the tightrope. *Emerg Med J.* 2005;22:612–616.
4. Opioid overdose. Bestpractice.bmj.com.

SECTION 11: PALLIATIVE CARE DRUG FORMULARY

PALLIATIVE CARE DRUG FORMULARY

Yee Choon Meng, Lee Hwei Khien, Christina Tan and Jade Wong

This table is intended as a quick point of care reference based on licensed and off-label indications and is not meant to be comprehensive. Please consult relevant drug references for more details or consult a pharmacist.

Drug	Route	Common Starting Dose	Max Daily Dose	Indications	Remarks
Alprazolam	PO	0.25 mg TDS*	10 mg	Anxiety.	
Amitriptyline	PO	10 to 25 mg ON*	150 mg (in divided doses)	Depression, neuropathic pain.	Use limited by anticholinergic and anti-alpha-adrenergic side effects. Anticholinergic side effects may be useful for sialorrhea in motor neuron disease (max 100 mg/day, off-label use).
Atropine sulfate 1% eye drops	SL	1 to 2 drops 6 H	2 to 4 drops 4 H	Excessive salivation, respiratory secretions.	Off-label use of eye drops for sublingual administration.
Bisacodyl (Dulcolax®)	PO	5 to 10 mg ON	60 mg	Constipation.	PO onset: 6 to 12 hrs.
	PR	10 to 20 mg daily			PR onset: 20 mins.

Calcitonin	SC/IM	4 units/kg BD	8 units/kg BD (if unsatisfactory response 48 hours after initiation).	Hypercalcemia of malignancy.	Usually reserved for rapid reduction of calcium levels (onset in 2 hours, effect diminishes after 48 hours).
Celecoxib	PO	100 mg BD	400 mg	Pain, inflammation.	
Chlorpromazine	PO	25 to 50 mg TDS 12.5 to 25 mg 6 H^	200 mg	Intractable hiccups. Nausea/vomiting.	Increases susceptibility to sunburn.
Clonazepam	PO	0.25 mg BD	4 mg	Anxiety.	
Codeine	PO	15 mg to 30 mg 4 H*	360 mg	Moderate pain.	
Denosumab (Xgeva®)	SC	120 mg ONCE 120 mg every 4 weeks		Hypercalcemia of malignancy. Prevention of skeletal related events in multiple myeloma and	May repeat dose after 7 days if hypercalcemia persists. May be considered for patients with renal impairment which limits use of bisphosphonates. May

(Continued)

(Continued)

Drug	Route	Common Starting Dose	Max Daily Dose	Indications	Remarks
				bone metastases from solid tumours.	lead to hypocalcemia in patients with CrCl <30 mL/min.
Dexamethasone	PO/SC/IV	4 to 8 mg daily	24 mg	Refractory nausea/vomiting, bone pain, hiccups.	Avoid dosing later than 2 pm to minimise sleep disturbance.
		6 to 16 mg daily		Bowel obstruction.	Consider prophylactic gastric protection in patients with previous peptic ulcer disease.
		8 to 16 mg daily		Raised intracranial pressure, lymphangitis carcinomatosis.	Do not stop abruptly if on >3 mg for >3 weeks, or if patient has a Cushingoid appearance.
		16mg daily		Superior vena cava obstruction, spinal cord compression.	

Drug	Route	Dose	Indication	Notes
Diazepam Enema	PR	10 to 20 mg PRN	Seizure.	PR onset: 5 to 10 mins.
Diclofenac	PO/PR IV/IM CSCI	25 mg TDS 75 mg PRN 75 mg over 24 hours	Bone pain, inflammation, fever.	Non-selective NSAID hence associated with an increased risk of GI events.
Domperidone	PO	10 mg TDS	Nausea/ vomiting, prokinetic.	HSA recommends a maximum dose of 30 mg/day due to risk of arrhythmias associated with higher doses.
Duloxetine	PO	30 to 60 mg daily	Depression.	May initiate at 30 mg daily. Increase after 1 week if patient able to tolerate.
		120 mg (in divided doses) No evidence of additional benefit for doses >60 mg/day	Neuropathic pain.	
Escitalopram	PO	5 to 10 mg OM*	Depression.	Lower risk of drug-drug interactions compared to other SSRIs.

(Continued)

(Continued)

Drug	Route	Common starting dose	Max daily dose	Indications	Remarks
Etoricoxib	PO	60 mg daily	120 mg	Pain, inflammation.	Limit use of 120 mg daily to 8 days.
Famotidine	PO/IV	40 mg daily	40 mg	Duodenal and non-malignant gastric ulcers, GERD, reflux esophagitis.	May increase to 40 mg BD for esophagitis.
Fentanyl Injection	SC	25 mcg 2 H PRN		Severe pain, dyspnea.	Conversion of parenteral:transdermal is 1:1.
	CSCI	10 mcg/hr			
Fentanyl Patch	Transdermal	6 mcg/hr every 72 hrs OR Convert from existing opioid at equianalgesic potency, changed every 72 hrs		Severe chronic pain.	Delayed onset — Do not use for management of acute or intermittent pain. When converting from CSCI, continue CSCI for up to 8 hours after initiation of patch. Converting from patch to CSCI: Remove patch and start CSCI at

Drug	Route	Dose	Max dose	Indication	Notes
					20% of existing patch dose. Increase CSCI to 120% of existing patch dose 8 hours after patch removed.
Fentanyl Sublingual Tablet (Abstral®)	SL	100 mcg, repeat 100 mcg after 30 mins if still in pain	800 mcg QDS PRN (at least 2 hrs apart)	Breakthrough cancer pain in opioid-tolerant patients.	Refer to Fentanyl chapter for information on dose titration. Do not switch from other fentanyl products at a 1:1 ratio.
Fluconazole	PO	100 mg daily for 7 to 14 days	200 mg	Moderate to severe oropharyngeal candidiasis.	For other indications, refer to drug monograph for dose regimens.
Gabapentin	PO	100 to 300 mg ON*	3600 mg	Neuropathic pain.	Start low and increase dose gradually based on response and tolerability.
		300 mg daily		Neuropathic or malignancy-related pruritus.	For uremic pruritus: If not on dialysis, use appropriate renal-adjusted dose.
		100 mg after hemodialysis	300 mg after hemodialysis	Uremic pruritus.	

(Continued)

(Continued)

Drug	Route	Common starting dose	Max daily dose	Indications	Remarks
Glycopyrronium	SC/IV	0.2 to 0.4 mg 4 H	2.4 mg	Respiratory and GI secretions, GI colic in bowel obstruction.	May have less effect on heart rate compared to Buscopan®. May reduce prokinetic effect of metoclopramide/domperidone.
	CSCI	0.6 to 2.4 mg over 24 hrs			
Haloperidol	PO	0.5 mg 6 H	20 mg	Agitation/delirium, nausea/vomiting, hiccups.	Avoid in Lewy Body Dementia CSCI: May not be very useful beyond 10 mg/day.
	SC/IM	1 to 2 mg 6 H			
	CSCI	2.5 to 10 mg over 24 hrs			
Hyoscine (Scopoderm®)	TD	1.5 mg (1 patch) every 72 hrs	3 mg every 72 hrs	Nausea/vomiting, respiratory secretions.	Apply patch behind ear Currently not registered in Singapore; stock availability may vary between institutions.
Hyoscine butylbromide (Buscopan®)	PO	10 mg TDS	100 mg	GI and genitourinary tract spasm.	

	SC/IV/IM	20 mg 6H	120 mg	Respiratory and GI secretions, GI colic in bowel obstruction.	
	CSCI	40 mg over 24 hrs			
Ibuprofen	PO	200 to 400 mg TDS (at least 4 hrs apart)	1200 mg	Pain, inflammation, fever.	Non-selective NSAID hence associated with an increased risk of GI events.
Ketamine	PO	10 to 25 mg TDS to QDS	200 mg	Neuropathic pain unresponsive to firstline analgesics, phantom limb or ischemic pain.	Use IV solution for oral administration. Dilute with flavored fluids to mask bitter taste.
	SC	10 to 25 mg PRN (0.5 mg/kg)			
	CSCI	Refer to Ketamine chapter			
Ketorolac	IV/IM	10 mg 4 H	90 mg (60 mg for elderly or weight <50 kg)	Bone pain, inflammation.	For short-term use not exceeding 3 weeks. For CSCI, dilute maximally with 0.9% saline as injection is irritant. Non-selective NSAID hence associated with an increased risk of GI events.
	CSCI	30 mg over 24 hrs			

(Continued)

(Continued)

Drug	Route	Common Starting Dose	Max Daily Dose	Indications	Remarks
Lactulose	PO	5 to 10 mL TDS	60 mL	Constipation.	May take 2 to 3 days to take effect. Adjust dose to achieve 2 to 3 soft stools per day.
Levetiracetam	PO/IV CSCI	250 mg BD 500 mg over 24 hrs	3000 mg	Hepatic encephalopathy. Seizures.	Conversion of PO:SC:IV is 1:1:1.
Lidocaine 5% plaster (Lignopad®)	Topical	1 plaster daily for 12 hrs within a 24 hr period	3 plasters	Neuropathic pain.	Allow a 12-hr plaster-free interval within a 24 hr period.
Lorazepam	PO/SL	0.5 to 1 mg daily*	10 mg	Insomnia, anxiety.	Use oral tablet for SL administration; SL formulation not available in Singapore.
Macrogol (Forlax®)	PO	1 sachet daily	8 sachets	Constipation.	Dissolve 1 sachet in at least 250mls of water. Associated with less flatulence than Lactulose.

Megestrol	PO	160 mg OM	800 mg	Anorexia/cachexia in cancer.	Stimulates appetite and weight gain; may take a few weeks to take effect.
Methadone			Refer to Methadone chapter		
Methylphenidate	PO	2.5 to 5 mg BD	40 mg	Depression in patients with short prognosis, fatigue, opioid-related drowsiness.	Dose no later than lunchtime to avoid insomnia Use immediate-release formulations.
Metoclopramide	PO/SC/IV/IM	10 mg TDS	1 mg/kg	Nausea/vomiting, prokinetic.	Avoid in complete bowel obstruction.
	CSCI	30 mg over 24 hrs			
Metronidazole	Topical	1 to 2 times daily		Odour control for fungating wounds.	Available as topical gel and 200 mg oral tablets. May crush oral tablets and sprinkle on wound (quantity of tablets depends on size of wound).

(Continued)

(Continued)

Drug	Route	Common Starting Dose	Max Daily Dose	Indications	Remarks
Midazolam	SC/IM/SL/Buccal	2 mg PRN	100 mg	Anxiety, agitation/delirium, seizure.	May be useful in intractable hiccups.
	CSCI	5 mg over 24 hrs			
Mirtazapine	PO	7.5 ON*	45 mg	Depression.	Exerts antidepressive effect in 1 to 2 weeks. Stimulates appetite Sedating at low doses (7.5 mg), may cause insomnia at high doses. Has anxiolytic effects.
Morphine	PO	2.5 mg 4 H PRN	No ceiling dose	Severe chronic pain, dyspnea.	May be converted to long-acting tablet when a stable regimen achieved.
	SC	2 mg 4H PRN			
	CSCI	0.2 mg/hr			
Nortriptyline	PO	10 mg ON*	150 mg	Depression, neuropathic pain.	

Nystatin suspension	PO	5 mL (500,000 units) QDS for 7 to 14 days	Mild oropharyngeal candidiasis.	Swish and retain in mouth as long as possible before swallowing.
Octreotide	SC	100 mcg TDS	900 mcg	Secretory diarrhea, reduce secretions in malignant intestinal obstruction.	Once control is established, may consider switching to maintenance therapy with IM depot (long-acting) injection.
	CSCI	200 mcg over 24hrs		
Olanzapine	PO/SL	2.5 mg ON or 2.5 mg 6H PRN	20 mg	Agitation/ delirium, nausea/vomiting.	Use orodispersible formulation for ease of administration.
Oxycodone	PO	5 mg 4 to 6H		Moderate to severe pain.	May be converted to long-acting tablet when a stable regimen achieved. Targin® (combination of oxycodone and naloxone) can be considered in patients with opioid-induced constipation despite laxative use.

(Continued)

(Continued)

Drug	Route	Common Starting Dose	Max Daily Dose	Indications	Remarks
Pamidronate	IV	15 to 90 mg depending on calcium levels		Hypercalcemia of malignancy.	Ensure patient is adequately hydrated before and during treatment. May repeat dose after 7 days if hypercalcemia persists. Limited data for dosing in severe renal impairment, consider alternative drugs.
		90 mg every 3 to 4 weeks		Bone pain.	
Paracetamol	PO	500 mg to 1000 mg, at least 4 hrs apart	4000 mg Patients at risk of hepatotoxicity: 2000 mg	Pain, fever.	
	PR	650 mg, at least 4 hrs apart	Patients ≤50 kg: 60 mg/kg not exceeding 3000 mg		

	Route	Dose		Indication	Notes
	IV	1000 mg, at least 4 hrs apart For patients ≤50 kg: 15 mg/kg, at least 4 hrs apart			
Paracetamol 500 mg + Codeine 8 mg (Panadeine®)	PO	2 tabs PRN, at least 4 hrs apart	8 tabs (or 4000mg of Paracetamol)	Pain.	
Parecoxib	IV/IM/SC	20 to 40 mg 12 H	80 mg (40 mg for elderly weighing <50 kg)	Bone pain, inflammation.	Limited clinical experience beyond 3 days.
	CSCI	40 mg over 24 hrs			
Phenobarbital	SC	100 mg 8 H	1600 mg	Seizures, terminal agitation refractory to other agents.	Dilute before administration to minimise site irritation Max daily doses up to 2400 mg have been used in palliative sedation.
	CSCI	400 mg over 24 hrs			

(Continued)

(Continued)

Drug	Route	Common Starting Dose	Max Daily Dose	Indications	Remarks
Pregabalin	PO	150 mg daily (in divided doses)	600 mg	Neuropathic pain.	Has anxiolytic effects. May be useful for refractory pruritus.
Prochlorperazine	PO IM	5 mg TDS 12.5 mg TDS	40 mg	Vertigo, nausea/vomiting.	Risk of local irritation prohibits SC administration.
Risperidone	PO	0.5 mg 6H	6 mg	Agitation/delirium, nausea/vomiting.	
Sennoside (Senna)	PO	7.5 to 15 mg ON	60mg	Constipation.	Onset: 8 to 12 hrs.
Sodium chloride 15% (Centa®) enema	PR	20 to 40 mL PRN		Constipation.	Preferred enema option in renal impairment as it does not contain phosphate.
Tramadol	PO	25 to 50 mg 8 H	400 mg	Moderate to severe pain.	

Tranexamic acid	PO	1000 mg TDS	4000 mg	Hemorrhage.	Use with caution in hematuria due to risk of clot retention in urinary tract.
	IV	500 mg TDS			
	Topical	500 mg		Surface bleeding.	Apply crushed tablet or gauze soaked in injection solution to bleeding site. For use as mouthwash, dissolve tablet in water and swirl in mouth.
Valproate (Epilim®)	PO	200 mg TDS	2500 mg (or 60 mg/kg/day)	Seizures, neuropathic pain.	Conversion of PO:SC is 1:1.
	CSCI	400 to 800 mg over 24 hrs (10 to 15 mg/kg/day)			
Venlafaxine	PO	37.5 to 75 mg OM	375 mg	Depression, anxiety, neuropathic pain.	Monitor for increased blood pressure.

(Continued)

(Continued)

Drug	Route	Common Starting Dose	Max Daily Dose	Indications	Remarks
Zoledronic acid (Zometa®)	IV	4 mg		Hypercalcemia of malignancy.	Ensure patient is adequately hydrated before and during treatment. May repeat dose after 7 days if hypercalcemia persists.
		4 mg every 3 to 4 weeks		Bone pain, prevention of skeletal related events.	

Collated with information from drug monographs and palliative care guidelines.

*Dose for elderly >65 years of age.

†Modified to accommodate local drug strengths.

INDEX

Printed in the United States
by Baker & Taylor Publisher Services